All About

Ketogenic Diet

Learn If this Diet is Right for You or NOT and What Food Options do You Have

Table of contents

INTRODUCTION

Fats, carbohydrates, and proteins are the three essential macronutrients responsible for a healthy body. Each of them has its special function to the body organs. For example, fats and carbohydrates are broken down to produce energy that helps in the body's physiological functions. In excess, these macronutrients might cause complications such as obesity and cancer. This occurs when you take more than the recommended amount of the nutrients.

Carbohydrates are the immediate sources of energy for the body. Excessive intake of sugars would mean the elevated insulin level to help in breaking down the carbohydrate for the production of energy. The fat in the diet is stored in the tissue resulting in the addition of weight.

Managing our diet is one way to enhance our health. The ketogenic diet is an ancient intervention that was used by the medical practitioners to enhance a metabolic state known as ketosis. This involves lipolysis as the primary source of energy. This recipe substitutes the carbohydrate with the fat as the primary source of energy. Because of the fat breakdown, ketones are produced to supply energy to the brain tissues. This causes a massive reduction in the insulin level as well as that of the blood sugar.

For two centuries, the low-carb diet has been helpful in the medical field. For example, John Rollo used it to manage diabetes among his patients. More than twenty clinical trials were conducted over the past eleven years to confirm the benefits of this diet.

Ketogenic diet differs from the low-carbohydrate diet. This is because the ketogenic diet replaces the neglected carbohydrate with the increased level of fat concentration. A low-carbohydrate recipe does not take into consideration the protein and fat composition.

Ketones are the by-products of restricted carbohydrate. It is important to determine the ketone bodies within your blood. There are home meters that are used to test the blood for the presence of ketones. Nova Max is an example of a company dealing with strip tests used for the determination of the blood ketone level. They are also able to test the blood glucose level.

It is important we consult our healthcare providers to advise us on the foods that comprise the ketogenic diet. Approximately, our keto diet should include 25% protein, 5% carbohydrates, and 70% fats. This will force the body to utilize the fat for energy at the expense of the carbohydrates. This, therefore, calls for our diet to contain the stated proportions.

Therapeutically, this program can be used for the long-term treatments of epilepsy, diabetes and reducing the seizures.

CHAPTER ONE: What is Ketogenic Diet?

When fat (one of the components of a good diet) accumulate in our bodies, a number of chronic conditions might result. Engaging in activities that would result in the breakdown of the fat is good for your general health. Since carbohydrates are the primary source of energy, reducing their intake will make the body burn the fat in return.

As a therapeutic program, physicians advice on the recipes that substitute the carbs with the fat as the main source of energy. Excluding one of the components of a diet might lead to nutritional disorders. The ketogenic diet, therefore, is a program that involves reducing the amount of sugar intake while increasing the fat consumption.

Keto diet has proven to be of great health benefits to the beneficiaries. Limiting the intake of glucose triggers the liver to break down the stored fat. This is lipolysis.

During ketosis, taking more starch will stimulate the secretion of the insulin by the β-cells. Insulin promotes the storage of fat in the adipocytes at the same time inhibits lipolysis. This is made possible by decreasing the process of adipose triglyceride lipase.

Breaking down fats produces ketones used in place of sugar as the source of energy within the body. Brain cells that require sugar for their functioning will turn to using the ketone bodies as their source of power.

A Brief History of ketogenic diet

For the idea of keto diet to be widespread, a number of personalities contributed towards its popularity. In the recent past, many people thought that consuming more fat was responsible for the addition of weight.

The idea of keto diet began long ago with an attempt to maintain a fit body shape and weight. This program is dated back to the late 17s when Dr. John Rollo published a book: *An Account of Two Cases of Diabetes Mellitus.* This book tried to explain his experience while trying to manage type 2 diabetes in his two patients. The patients were subjected to diet with less amount of carbohydrates and increased amount of fat and moderate protein level. In this period, there was no proven medication for the diabetic conditions.

In the year 1863, William Banting published the *On Corpulence* following his struggle to fight obesity. He tried to explain the miraculous transformation of Dr. Harvey's intervention. Dr. Harvey wanted to experiment the low-carb diet as an intervention for obesity having returned from a convention in Paris on the new dietary means of controlling this condition. Banting is referred as the Early Champion of Low-carb Diet since he promoted the intervention through his publications. He followed the diet until his death, but his teachings are still with us.

To date, the Mayo Clinic promoted the work of Mr. Banting by putting their clients on a low-carb diet until they achieve their desired weight. This program includes two phases: "the lose it!" and "the live it!" The main principle behind this intervention was to lose pounds of kilojoules as you aim at improving your livelihood. Pioneers of Mayo Clinic Diet are not restrictive on the type of food you take. Vegetarians should see no problem in the Mayo plan.

The application of this diet as an intervention was broadly recognized in the 1920s to treat epilepsy. In the late 19's, Jim Abraham's son used the innovation to treat his epileptic conditions. This made it common to date.

CHAPTER TWO: Ketogenic vs. Low-carb Diet

As mentioned earlier, it is important we consume all the important components of a diet: fat, carbohydrate, and protein. A disorder might occur if correct proportions of these constituents are not maintained.

The increase in weight is associated with the uncontrolled intake of sugar within the body. When the sugar is let into the body, it is broken down to produce energy that facilitates the proper functioning of the body organs. As a result, the fat included in the diet is stored in the body tissues. This is responsible for the additional weight among the affected. The addition of body mass predisposes the individuals to chronic conditions like the heart diseases.

To control the rising cases of chronic diseases, medical practitioners implement various interventions that aim at managing these accelerating incidences. This rose as a concern after the subjects tried starving themselves in order to lose weight. Considering the connection between a lot of carbohydrates and chronic conditions, physicians thought of carb-restriction as a mean of managing the undesirable states.

Though the fats are an important component of the diet, avoiding the hydrogenated ones is important since they are highly linked to the chronic heart conditions.

The restricted intake of starch ensures that the fat in the diet is utilized as the primary source of energy within the body. With this, two types of diets were identified: ketogenic and the low-carb diets. It is difficult to note the difference between the two. This calls for special knowledge and Visiting a qualified physician before opting for what you believe to be a ketogenic diet.

Special differences between the ketogenic and low-carb diet.

A low-carb diet is evidenced when about 150 grams (half the normal amount) of sugar is consumed according to the typical American diet. Further cutting the intake of fat to less than 50 grams in a day is common for those trying to shift to ketosis.

Unlike in the normal low-carb diet, keto diet ensures the intake of moderate amount of proteins to perform their primary function. This extra consumption of fat replaces the cut carb as the primary source of energy.

To understand the difference between the two diet types, below are some of the critical facts to consider:

1. Some calories provided to the body.

The difference between the two types of diets depends on the percentage of carbohydrate. Though the intention of both diets is to reduce the amount of this macro nutrient, the composition in low-carb is higher (40% calories) than in the keto diet (5% calories). Physicians advise their patients on the low-carb recipes to let them feed their specific dosha.

2. Replacement of lost calories

Both strategies aim at restricting the consumption of carbohydrates (the primary source of energy). The only difference between the two is that in the normal low-carb diet the lost calories are not replaced. Keto diet, on the other hand, replaces the carbohydrates with fat to act as the reliable source of energy. This maintains the body in a metabolic state called ketosis. The ketone bodies produce the desired energy to the brain cells and other body cells.

3. Composition of the other components in a diet

Reducing the amount of starch will not be beneficial if not controlled. A specific ratio between the three common components: the carbohydrate, protein, and fat must be maintained. The fact that the low-carb recipe does not interfere with the fat and protein ratios upon reducing the proportion of the carbohydrate makes it different from ketogenic meals.

 In ketogenic diets, the reduced consumption of sugar is substituted with an increased amount of fat. Protein has to be included in the moderate amount. The fat is broken down to ketones that provide the needed fuel.

4. The ultimate body state

The major difference between these two types of diet is the ultimate metabolic state of the body. Ketogenic diets ensure that the ketone bodies resulting from the fat breakdown are the primary sources of energy for the brain and other body cells.

 In those under the low-carb diet, the fewer carbohydrates are still the primary energy source. A state of ketosis is not experienced with this type of recipe.

5. Sodium electrolyte

Reducing the amount of sugar in your diet will mean that the level of insulin drops. The drop in insulin level will lead to the excessive shedding of sodium by the kidney. Sodium, therefore, should be added into the diet upon restricting the carbohydrate intake.

In ketogenic, as opposed to the normal low-carb diet, the sodium supplements are added to the diet to substitute the functions of the insulin hormone. The low-carb recipe does not consider the effect of lowering the hormone level.

The main aim of restricting the intake of sugar into the body can either be treating conditions like epilepsy or controlling obesity. In a ketogenic diet, the other components of a meal are balanced to ensure the body functions are promoted.

Cutting the intake of carbohydrate does not necessarily mean that your body is in ketosis state. Adding an extra amount of fat in your diet will ensure the body cells use ketone bodies as the powerhouse.

In the low-carb diets, the amount of protein is not monitored. Increased amount of protein in the meal might lead to gluconeogenesis: turning the extra amino acids to glucose. The glucose will then be utilized as the source of energy.

CHAPTER THREE: How to Test Your Blood for Ketones

Your body is said to be in ketosis when it uses ketones as fuel for the brain and other body cells. This occurs when you reduce the intake of carbs and increase that of fat. This insignificant amount of glucose in diet will shift the body to begin utilizing the fat.

Shifting your body to depend on fat as the source of power at the expense of the sugar has several health benefits like cutting down extra weight that predisposes one to other chronic conditions. Taking keto diet requires the physicians' involvement. The professionals strive to ensure their clients meet the ultimate health goal.

Too little amount of ketones within the body will shift the body from utilizing the fat to using the carbs as the energy source. Again, very high concentration of these fuel components will acidify the blood, a condition called ketoacidosis.

Regular testing of both the blood and urine for the presence of the ketones is recommended. Testing urine is not recommended since it is believed to give the counts of the excess ketones excreted. A blood test is, therefore, the most preferred.

Different ways to test your ketone concentration

Different criteria are available for testing the three different types of ketone bodies: Beta-Hydroxybutyrate (BHB), Acetone and Acetoacetate. It is not easy to detect the fluctuating concentration of the ketones within the blood channels.

For the estimation of your ketone counts, consider either of the following means to ensure you remain in ketosis:

✓ Blood ketone meter

A basic blood ketone tester has two basic components: *lancet pen* that helps in drawing a blood sample from the individual and the *test strips* (the most expensive part of the device).

There are different brands of the ketone test devices from different manufacturers. They come at varying prices to favor the different economic status of the users. Some of the dominating testers include the Precision and the Nova Max brands.

The ketone meter is only reliable when measuring the concentration of the BHB ketone bodies.

✓ Breath of acetone

Acetones might result due to decarboxylation of the acetoacetate. This acetone is responsible for the sweet odor in a breath when in ketosis. This is also a way of determining whether your body is in ketosis. This can be detected in your urine, sweat or even the breath.

However, this helps you determine whether your body is in ketosis, it is said that the breath ketones might be affected by several factors like alcohol consumption.

Steps involved in the testing of the ketone bodies concentration.

The blood examination about the composition of ketone bodies should follow a specific procedure. This should be systematically trailed. The procedure is similar to that involved in blood sugar testing.

- Before you get hold of the testing device, it is important you wash your hands with soap and ensure you dry them appropriately.

- The next step is to load a sterilized needle into the lancet pen. Steps to follow while placing the needle is included in the package and should be followed keenly to avoid any inconveniences.

- Once the lancet is in place, remove the blood ketone strip from its package and fix it into the meter brand of your choice. This should be done carefully to ensure you get the correct reading of your ketone concentration.

- Carefully prick your finger to draw blood from the veins. This is made possible by placing the pen on one side of the fingertip then pushing the lancet button. This will allow an opening for blood to come out before it is let into the strip.

- To allow accurate result, the size of the blood drop will vary from one meter to another. This call for gentle pressing of the pricked finger to force it to produce enough amount of blood needed for the test.

- Once you have enough blood, fill the ketone strip. This is done by allowing the end of the strip to touch the produced blood drop. This is given time until the little openings, and the meter registers are filled.

- After the blood covers the test strip, let it be undisturbed for a few seconds before reading the result. Record the result then interpret it well to have a clear picture of your blood-ketone composition. . Like earlier indicated, interpreting the result varies depending on whether you are having the test for ketoacidosis determination or you are on a keto diet.

- Safely dispose of both the used lancet and test strip. This will enhance the safety of the public as a requirement by the public health department. The disposal is somehow segregated since the lancet is disposed into the sharp bin with the other sharps.

For those who are in normal ketosis, the normal ketone count in the serum should range between **0.5 and 3.0 mM**.

Timing the blood ketone testing

Depending on the time of the day, the ketone concentration varies. For example, the level is always highest during the morning hours after an overnight fast. This means that the test should be done on a specific time of the day daily (for example taking the test at 8 am every day). This helps to track the best comparison of the fluctuating level of the ketone bodies with the different conditions of the day.

On the contrary, for those with the types 1 and 2 diabetes or drunks, ketone testing can be conducted at any time of the day due to the fear of ketoacidosis.

Important precautions when taking the blood ketone test.

1. Before using the strip, it is important you confirm the expiry date. The out of date test strips will produce inaccurate results.

2. Before purchasing a test strip, ensure you buy the test strip that corresponds to your selected meter brand. This is because they are not substitutable.

It is important you determine your blood ketone concentration regularly. Follow the correct procedure to get accurate results. Have knowledge on the interpretation of your findings. There are many brands of ketone meters to meet your individualized taste.

A specific time for the test should be identified in case it is for nutritional purpose. For the ketoacidosis detection, the test can be done anytime of the day to give reliable outcomes.

CHAPTER FOUR: Best Foods for Ketogenic Diet

Food is essential for our body's growth and development. On the contrary, what we eat can at times be disastrous to our health. With this, we can conclude that being in any diet is not an easy program as it sounds. This is because feeding takes into consideration many factors including the specific body types.

The desire to live a healthy life with ketosis has made many people turn to a ketogenic diet for help. This diet takes into account the cutting off carbohydrate intake. Unlike the Atkins diet, keto diet substitutes the carbs with the fat as the primary source of energy. The other three components of a diet are included in this keto diet in proportions that would maintain the body physiological processes.

The proportion of the fats, carbohydrates, and proteins in a diet will vary from one individual to the other.

Food sources of the three basic macronutrients for ketosis

For keto diet, all the three macronutrients must be consumed. Different foods are known to be the sources of the ketogenic macronutrients. Having knowledge on the ketogenic diet will ensure you go for foods that are whole and offer the best nutrition. Processed foods might contain additives that are harmful to the health of an individual.

Ketogenic foods have special properties that help in maintaining the body in the state of ketosis. These properties must be taken into consideration:

1. Energy density- foods with high concentration of water and fiber levels normally have a low energy density. This makes us full with the fewer calories we consume.

2. Nutrient density- one importance of ketogenic dishes is that it prevents cravings. Foods with high nutrients density will not only satisfy the consumer with fewer calories but also avoid the undesirable craving.

3. Insulin load- insulin is vital in breaking down the carbohydrates for the production of energy within the body. Replacing the starch with fat means that the insulin hormone will have no significant role during the digestion.

 Therefore considering the non-starchy foods with high insulinogenic calories is good for the lovers of ketosis. This is because they have low insulin load per 100g of food. The food will have to be consumed in large amount to affect the insulin significantly.

4. Net carbohydrate- foods rich in carbohydrates are replaced with those high in fat content. The less concentration of the carb included in the diet helps in leveling the blood glucose.

5. Percentage of insulinogenic calories- These energies require insulin to process.

Before deciding on the parameters above in the keto diet, consider your blood-glucose level and your goal to lose weight.

Some examples of foods for the ketogenic diet

In a ketogenic diet, fats are the primary sources of energy. Cutting down the amount of starch, which is the ultimate source of energy within the body, leads to the need to increase the fat intake.

Depending on the individual's type of digestion, the fats can be dangerous hence the need to consult a qualified physician before opting for the roles of fats in ketosis. Choosing the right fats for your diet is very vital. For example, fat from whole foods is the best to consider.

The Omega-3and Omega-6 are essential fatty acids in our body and should be included in our diet. These essential nutrients are found in different foods and hence the need to introduce all the sources in our diet.

For example, avocado and kale are some of the sources of the Omega-3 fatty acids while the pumpkin seeds and the raw sunflower seeds are some of the foods rich in Omega-6 fatty acids.

In addition to the increased fat concentration and the cut carb levels, moderate amount of proteins enhance ketosis. With all the diet components and in their correct composition, the organic foods are more preferred for ketotic individuals. The following foods are important for ketosis:

a. Fish

The wild fish like the salmon and shellfish enhances a balance of the Omega-3 fatty acids. Supplementing significant amount of fish oil will be great for those who are not lovers of the aquatic inhabitant.

b. Eggs

Eggs are the foods considered by the diabetics and those on ketogenic diets. This is because they have a low carbohydrate concentration. The egg yolk is chemically stable.

c. Avocado

Avocado can be eaten in any phase of Atkins. The fat in the avocado will enhance the production of ketones that acts as the alternative sources of energy. With this food, your hunger is at bay and the craving satisfied.

d. Nuts

Nuts like the macadamia nuts have the healthy fats and the nutrients such as the vitamin E. The high-energy property of this product, and its tasty nature makes the users consume more than the desired amount. Nuts have about 74% fat compared to the 13% carbohydrates.

e. Meat (not lean meat)

Beef, goat, lamb and the wild game that feed on grass are known to have the recommended fatty acid counts.

f. Pork

Pork products like the pork loins and the ham are important foods to include in your keto diet. The added sugars of the ham should also be monitored to prevent it from being broken down at the expense of the ketones in keto diet.

g. Poultry

Poultry like the chickens, quails and the pheasant that are not fed from processed foods. The free rangers are preferred to the commercial ones.

h. Dairy products

For this keto diet, the raw and organic milk products are the best dairy products to be considered. Cheese and the cream are used to provide ketogenic meals that will help you attain your goal for ketosis.

i. Vegetables

The green leafy vegetables that are grown on the surface are the ones preferred in keto diet. Though both the organic and non-organic greens have the same nutritive importance, those that are treated with chemicals might poison the user.

Choosing the vegetables with less sugar but high in nutrients is important in the keto diet and therefore those with high sugar should be excluded. The leafy ketogenic foods that fall under the same class with kale or spinach are ketogenic.

j. Beverages

The natural diuretic effects of the keto diet make dehydration a common experience. Rehydration is, therefore, vital in ensuring we maintain our bodies' physiological processes. Consuming liquids like the coffee, water, and tea will help in replacing the lost water.

k. Sweeteners

To achieve the goal of the ketogenic diet, it is important to cut off the sweet foods from your daily feedings. This is because they are known to accelerate the concentration of sugar in our body.

The sweeteners that lack either or both the dextrose and maltodextrin should be consumed for ketosis. This is because they have some content sugar. Most liquid sweeteners like the stevia and Erythritol are the preferred for the achievement of ketosis since they lack the dextrose and maltodextrin binders. So here is a quick list of sweeteners you can include for your well-deserved dessert:

Xylitol: Is about two-thirds of the caloric value of regular white sugar, so it contains 2.5 calories per gram, so it is not completely non-caloric. Therefore, you need to watch out when you are following the Keto-diet more so than the Low-carb diet.

Yacon Syrup: This natural syrup is extracted from the Yacon plant that naturally grows in the Andes of South America. It is high in complex carbohydrates called fructooligosaccharides (about 50% FOS or Fructooligosacharides) that function as soluble fibers which feed the intestinal microbiome. Yacon syrup has little effect in increasing the blood glucose.

Erythritol: it is a sugar alcohol, and its caloric value is between 6% and 8% of the calories as white sugar, and it tastes less sweet as well somewhere 60-80% of the sweetness. This is another sweetener that you need to use in small amounts since it can affect your blood glucose and can take you out of Ketosis.

Stevia: This plant is native to South America, and Paraguay in particular. This plant is not only used for its sweetness taste but also for its medicinal value. Stevia is very sweet, but its caloric value almost does not exist so it makes it very Ketogenic friendly sweetener.

I. Spices

Most spices have very little carbs. Manufacturers add more sugar to their products as fillers and therefore their consumption should be monitored. When in the ketogenic diet, it is important to read the labels of the spices before their use to identify any added sugar. For example, sea salt and the black pepper are the best spices to add to your recipe.

Fats and Oils: this is not an exhaustive list but you will sufficient number of choices.

-Extra Virgin Olive Oil

-Butter

-Lard

-Duck and Goose Fat

-Tallow

-Coconut Oil

-Red Palm Oil

-Ghee

-Moderate amount of Sesame Oil

- Moderate amount of Avocado Oil

-Moderate amount of Flaxseed Oil

-Small amount of other seed/vegetable oils since you will get polyunsaturated fatty acids from whole foods such as vegetables, nuts, and legumes.

Precaution

Most foods, even those that are consumed to enhance ketosis contain natural sugars. It is, therefore, important to regulate their usage to achieve your goal of ketosis. Let your qualified physician who's knowledgeable about ketogenic and low-carb diets to guide you towards your ketogenic journey.

CHAPTER FIVE: Ketogenic diet for fast weight loss

From a non-professional perspective, the addition of weight is linked to the excessive intake of fat. This condition contributes to the increased incidences of chronic conditions like the obesity and sometimes heart dysfunctions.

Addition of weight is associated with the increased intake of carbohydrates. Elevated intake of sugar will cause the fluctuation of the blood sugar levels and hence high production of insulin. As a result, the lipids are stored within the body tissues making the affected exposed to chronic conditions like the heart diseases.

Interventions to cut some extra weight have been proven helpful in controlling the chronic issues. Among the many programs involved in losing weight for healthy living, ketosis is one of the recommended processes. Ketosis is the process by which the body breaks down the ketones for the production of energy for the proper functioning of the brain cells and other body organs.

This ketosis state is achieved by an individual relying on a ketogenic diet. This recipe involves cutting down the intake of carbs and replacing it with fat. Unlike in normal low-carb diet, keto diet further reduces the percentage of sugar intake to about 5% the total composition. This, as said earlier, ensures that the body replaces the breakdown of sugar with the fats. In addition to the added composition of fats, moderate amount of proteins is also maintained.

Reducing the number of carbohydrates will mean that the production of insulin is minimized causing the body to alternatively turn on breaking down the fat as the primary source of energy. Adapting your body to the state of ketosis is a gradual process that sometimes makes one experience the feeling of withdrawal. The fat that was stored in the different body tissues will be broken down thereby reducing the extra weight.

In keto diet, the small amount of sugar added is responsible for the special muscle development and alignment. The protein component must be moderate on the ketogenic diet since excess protein will facilitate gluconeogenesis hence continued breakdown of glucose as the source of energy.

Special Tips into ketosis for weight loss

- Consuming less protein is critical

With the aim of cutting down weight while in the ketogenic diet, the stored fat is broken down to produce the needed energy. In keto diet, it is important to ingest the moderate amount of protein to help in the body's physiological processes.

Taking excess protein will interfere with ketosis since it might stimulate the **gluconeogenesis**. This ensures the continuous metabolism of the carbs as the primary source of energy. This will lead to accumulation of fats at the tissues hence added mass.

- Eat more fat (Mostly Monounsaturated and Saturated fats)

In keto diet inclusion of fat is a necessity and not a side item. Foods rich in fat such as the avocados and the egg yolks must be included in the ketogenic diet. Selection of the good fats from the bad fats is important.

Increased intake of fat will mean that they become the primary sources of energy within the body. The ketones will supply the needed energy to the brain cells. This will, as a result, lead to the reduced weight to meet your desired body shape.

- Limit the intake of carbs

Ketosis means that your body uses the ketone bodies as the primary sources of power. Therefore, carbohydrate is not needed in a large amount in a keto diet. About 5% the total diet components are enough to ensure the fats are the ones broken down and as a result cutting down the undesirable extra weight.

The important point in keto diet is replacing the cut carbs with extra fat to maintain the body functioning.

- Regular blood ketone testing

A blood ketone meter will help you test your blood for ketone to confirm that the fat is the one broken down as the source of energy. Though the testers are normally not accurate, they give an overview of the ketone blood state. In ketosis, the higher a number of ketones in the blood, the better.

This will ultimately reduce the extra weight of the one under the ketogenic diet. Excess ketones lead to a condition ketoacidosis and hence the need to constantly monitor its concentration.

- Consider a fat fast.

For a body to be in ketosis, it takes time for it to adapt. It is important to go for a fat fast. This ensures your body get used to the new system. This will ensure your body will begin using the fat as the primary sources of energy for the body cells. With this, you can be sure that you lose the extra weight that makes your life unbearable for you. I do suggest you do that gradually with small increments of fat especially if you have been following a low-fat diet for some time.

- Keto-diet Ratio

Eating the correct amount of food every day is good for maintaining a ketosis state of the body. This will ensure you do not consume the extra amount of protein that might lead to gluconeogenesis, which might negatively affect ketosis. The best thing with this is that when you are on this diet, it naturally reduces hunger. The ratio for many individuals should be 4:1 which means for every four grams of fat you consume you should have no more than 1 gram of carbohydrates and protein.

- Having patience

To kick start ketosis, time is required after introducing the high fat diet. This is because initially the body was used to metabolizing carbs as a source of energy.

About two to three weeks will be great in ensuring your system fully adapts to this state.

- Being optimistic of attaining your desired body shape

Ketosis involves balancing the cortisol, ghrelin and leptin hormones. Visualizing your body when in good shape to trigger your brain and the hormones in the process. This ruling out of negative thoughts will ensure you live a stress-free lifestyle that promotes ketosis and ultimately help in cutting down on extra weight.

CHAPTER SIX: Keto Diet for Individuals with Special Needs

Neurological diseases such as the Parkinson disease and the epilepsy are on the rise regardless of the many pharmacological interventions implemented in the fight against such conditions.

The diseases possess pathological effects to the general physiological processes of the body. Combining ketogenic foods as a form of medication with the other normal anticonvulsant medication has proven to be one of the special measures in children.

To experience the positive outcomes of this diet as a therapeutic remedy, a medical team consisting of a dietician and a neurologist ensure that the side effects that might occur as a result are controlled. This will help the affected define the absolute ketogenic diet that would help in retrieving their normal health. The blood of the subject is analyzed before deciding whether to subject him or her to ketogenic foods as a way to his or her recovery.

Among the many ill conditions that can be managed by following a keto diet, epilepsy, seizure, and diabetes are some of the conditions that are discussed in this special publication. In case you are experiencing or have a loved one suffering from such, special information on the importance of this intervention will help your body recover from the crisis.

Ketogenic Diet for Epilepsy

The difficult-to-control type of epilepsies like the Lennox-Gastaut is associated with severe convulsion. This usually occurs in individuals with neurological issues. This facilitates ketone bodies production within the blood channels. This lessens the occurrences of seizures.

Considering the Atkins ideology on the use of high-fat diet to control epileptic conditions, many people tried to experiment this cheap management procedure. Unfortunately, the intervention that was thought to be the long-awaited remedy against this demon lost favor in the eyes of its lovers. This was because the beneficiaries failed to follow the diet plan and hence the elevating cholesterol levels.

In the year 2008, a new trial was conducted on the hypothesized benefits of the once neglected keto diet as a remedy against epilepsy. It was realized that this diet alters the brain metabolism. This in return help in minimizing the occurrence of seizures. The positive outcome of this research rekindled the favor in its use. The diet is easy to follow to experience its health benefits in that particular aspect.

The epileptics must first be hospitalized for the medical practitioners to monitor their progress for the initial stages of this intervention. According to the professionals, it is recommended that the sick go for about two days without taking any food before kicking off this recovery progress. This diet lacks the essential vitamins and hence must be supplemented with the processed sugar-free vitamin.

Consequentially, those under this diet as a remedy for this neurological disorder will not be able to grow effectively or even add weight during this period. Monitoring this process is important to allow for a normal growth after ketosis.

How monitoring is done during this time

> ➤ Maintaining the correct weight

When using this strategy to manage epilepsy, the individuals do not add weight. In case they add mass, the dietician is required to adjust their clients' diet.

> ➤ Regular blood and urine tests

Ketosis means that fat is broken as the primary source of energy. Ketones are produced as a result. Analyzing both the blood and urine to measure the amount of ketones available should be made a necessity. Significant ketones count will mean that there is no medical issue. If the count is minimal, then it signifies that the body still breaks down the carbs instead of the fat.

> ➤ Anthropometric measurements

One indicator that our body is in ketosis is the slowed growth. The height and weight are measured regularly to determine this state.

> ➤ The medical practitioner will always check on their patients every 1-3 months to detect any undesirable state of the body during this period.

If the strategy is effective, one should be subjected to the diet for about two years. Immediately after the patient fully recovers from the epileptic attack, it is advisable to get out of the diet since when a person stays on a diet for a longer period of time, then some side effects arises. Some of the side effects that are associated with this include the following:

- Elevated cholesterol levels- this is usually linked to consumption of bad fat such as partially hydrogenated oils and highly processed seed/vegetable oils. To avoid this, early evacuation from the diet will be helpful.

- Kidney stones

- Constipation

- Slowed weight gain and growth

- Weak bones that manifest as fracture

- Dehydrations

- Reduced blood sugar level

- Frequent vomiting

When should one turn to ketogenic diet as a way to control seizure and epilepsy as a result?

Professionals are preferred to subject the sick to a ketogenic diet. Before this, a number of criteria must be met before opting for the benefits of this intervention.

❖ One must have tried two or three anti-seizure medications in vain before jumping to this dietary option as the ultimate solution. In some cases, it can be considered as the first choice intervention.

- ❖ The caregivers of the sick must understand the therapy inside out. This will enable them to support the dietary therapy and as a result help in the management of epilepsy.
- ❖ Once the caretakers get to know all about the diet, they have to commit to it for at least three months before beginning to observe its effects.
- ❖ The ability to control the side effects that might occur when in this diet. For example the basic management of nausea.

Ketogenic Diet for Diabetes

Diabetes is a condition that is related to the elevated blood sugar levels. The increase in blood sugar level can be because of the pancreas failure to produce enough insulin or the body cells inability to respond to the insulin produced. This leads to the two types of diabetes: type 1 and type 2. The third type of diabetes called gestational diabetes is common during the pregnancy period.

The type 2 diabetes is the most common of the disease types. This normally affects the big bodied. Many strategies have been developed to contain the ailment. Insulin injection or tablets are commonly used as the remedy.

In the early days before the introduction of insulin supplements, professional health practitioners advised on the importance of keto diet in the management of diabetes. Ketogenic diet maintains the body in ketosis. This means that the fat broken down at the expense of sugar produces ketone bodies that are helpful in supplying the desired energy within the body.

Since the body systems of those suffering from type 2 diabetes does not respond to the insulin produced, the sugar concentration within the blood increases. Relying on high-fat diets with low-carbs is seen as a remedy since there will be less starch within the body hence maintaining the elevating glucose level. This will also minimize insulin resistance among those suffering from the type 2 condition.

The minimum level of carbs for those with type 2 diabetes

Regardless of the health condition, everyone requires a certain percentage of sugar that is vital for the normal functioning of his or her body system.

In estimation, the lowest count of carbs per day should be 40 grams that are equivalent to about 180 calories. This means that those under the ketogenic diet should not completely cut the ingestion of carbs. A little sugar will at least facilitate the absorption of the amino acids from the blood channel.

Subjecting yourself to ketogenic diet should only be done under professional supervision to avoid the resultant side effects. Nonetheless, being under ketogenic diet will bid goodbye to the diabetic drugs, insulin, and diabetes forever.

Does ketogenic diet reduces Seizures [1]

Epileptic attacks are linked to the development of seizures. Therefore, the ability of this keto diet to manage epilepsy is enough to prove that it reduces the occurrences of seizure. Seizures, just like epilepsy, greatly affects the quality of life.

This attack occurs when one cell fires uncontrollably thereby affecting the other neighboring cells. This is one of the common manifestations of epilepsy in individuals. This is because the energy production within our brain cells is altered due to certain unhealthy lifestyles like living an inactive lifestyle among other causes.

Keto diet is one of the long-term management of seizures that affects the health of the brain. The ketone bodies produced by the breakdown of fat will provide the energy required for the brain cell functioning.

CHAPTER SEVEN: Ketogenic Diet Recipes for Meals and Snacks

The health benefits of the low-carb diets cannot be underestimated. Consumption of the foods high in fat but with low carbohydrates fully explains the keto diet. This diet, unlike the Atkins, does recognize the nutritional value of carbohydrates. This means that they are not completely excluded from the daily meal.

Medical practitioners and the dieticians have recommended several combinations of the ketogenic foods known as a recipe. The unique recipes are to be followed strictly for our body to gain the ketosis state.

The epileptic and those with the type 2 diabetes rely on the unique therapeutic properties of these foods. The high fat concentration replacing the cut sugar can reduce the occurrence of a seizure.

Vegetarians are those individuals whose system do not accommodate the non-vegetable food components. This makes it a special subject to discuss since it most of the ketogenic foods are products from the animal. For example, butter, whole milk, and the red meat. A small amount of vegetable oils can also be of help in maintaining the utilization of ketone bodies as the primary sources of energy.

Simple ketogenic recipes to maintain your body in ketosis

Keto diet was earlier regarded as unappetizing, unappealing and boring. Professional nutritionists illustrate different mouth-watering snacks and meals.

All the recipes recommended by the dieticians have the following characteristics:

❖ The calories count must be accounted for in the diet. The meals have to be keto approved. This means that the overall components of the diet must have significantly reduced the amount of carb and high-fat amount.

❖ Include the diet component in its correct proportions. The 4:1 ratio of the fat to carbs will ensure that the body utilizes the fats as the primary energy source rather than the sugar.

❖ The recipe has to be denoted to specify their targets. For example, "vegetarian" to mean that it is recommended for the vegetarians.

Oven-Fried Coconut Chicken Drumsticks

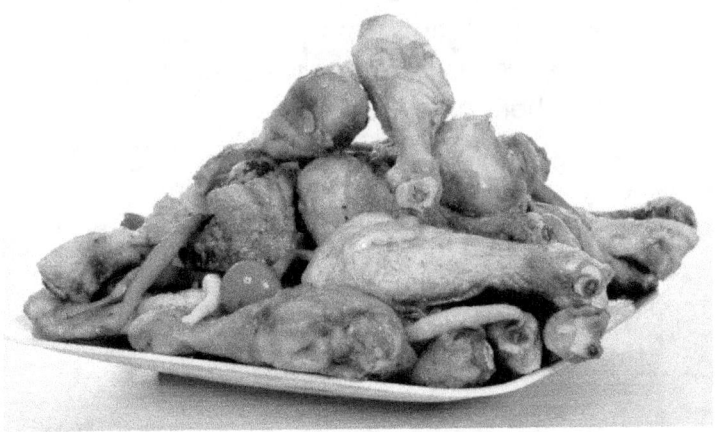

For the lovers of the coconut flavor, this oven fried coconut chicken drumsticks is the best chicken recipe for you. This high-fat low-carb meal is recommended for those whose bodies are in ketosis.

Requirements

- ➢ 2 eggs
- ➢ 12 chicken drumsticks
- ➢ 1 cup of coconut flour
- ➢ 1 cup of unsweetened shredded coconut
- ➢ Two tablespoons of coconut oil

Preparation for this recipe

1. The first step is to preheat the oven to about 400 degrees Celsius
2. In a bowl, whisk the two eggs lightly
3. Mix the shredded coconut and the coconut flour in a bowl.

4. Each of the 12 drumsticks is dipped in the whisked egg then finally in the coconut mixture.
5. Place a pan in the oven to slightly heat before melting the 2 tablespoons of the coconut oil.
6. Fry each drumstick for about 2 minutes before placing them on a wire rack.
7. In an oven, place the wire rack containing the drumsticks for a minimum of 40 minutes
8. After the 40 minutes, it is advisable to let the drumstick rest for a maximum of 10 minutes. This will allow the juices in the meat to settle.
9. The meal is ready for only 4 serves

Homemade Italian Meatballs made with Grass Fed Ground Beef

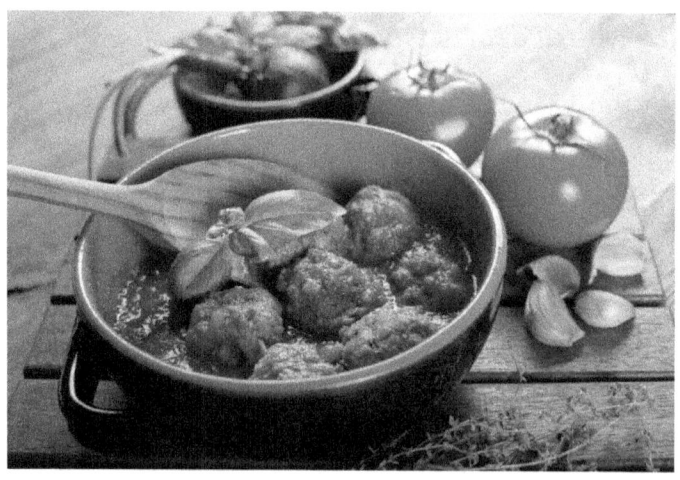

In this recipe, the main ingredient is the beef from the grass fed animals. The beef has to be ground.

Grinding is proven to reduce the quality of meat as well as chances of bacterial infection.

The homemade tomato sauce from the organic tomatoes has to be prepared before the recipe preparation. The industrial sauce contains many additives that might have side effects to the health of the user.

This recipe is ideal for all occasions.

Ingredients

- 1 egg
- ¼ cup of almond flour
- ¼ teaspoon of pepper
- ½ teaspoon salt
- 3 tablespoon of homemade tomato sauce
- ¾-cup sharp cheddar cheese for topping.
- ½ cup sharp cheddar cheese for mixture
- 1 packet of grass fed ground beef
- 2 tablespoon of butter from grass fed animals. This is for frying
- 1 teaspoon Italian seasoning

Recipe preparation

1. In a large mixing bowl, mix the ground beef, almond flour, egg, pepper, salt, Italian seasoning, tomato sauce and the ½ a cup of the cheese.
2. After a fine mixture is achieved, roll up the meatballs to suit your preference. This is in terms of numbers and the meatball size.

3. Preheat the pan over medium heat then melt the butter in the pan.
4. Into the melted butter, add the already rolled meatballs then allow them to pan-fry for about 4 minutes on both sides.
5. On a broiler-proof pan, top each of the beef rolls with the remaining ¾-cup cheese.
6. Put the cheese-topped meat rolls under the broiler for about a minute.
7. After the timed minute, the meal is ready to serve four places.

Depending on the size of the beef balls, regulate the cooking time. For example, larger balls will require more time to cook.

Organic tomato source is preferred to those from the supermarket, which has added sugar and other additives.

Three Cheese Bacon Tomato Frittata

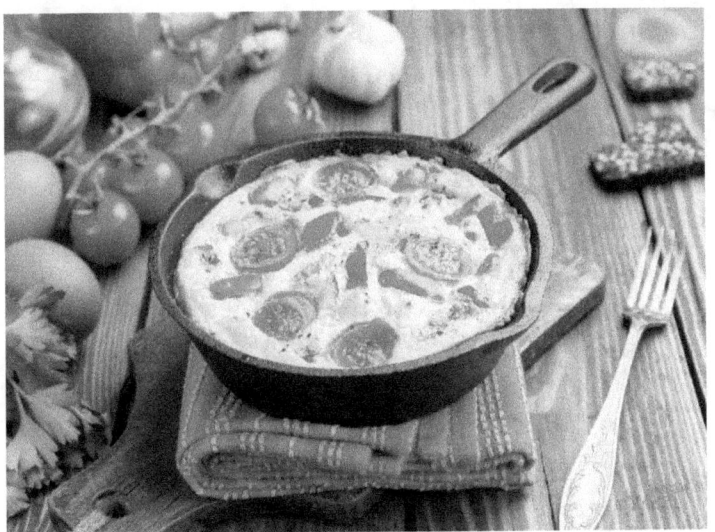

Starting a day for those under ketogenic diet is enhanced by taking this meal for breakfast. Prepared frittata meal can last for a maximum of 3 days if stored well in a refrigerator.

Ingredients

- ➢ 6 slices of bacon
- ➢ 1 cup of cherry tomatoes
- ➢ 10 eggs
- ➢ ¼ cup of heavy cream
- ➢ ¼ a cup of parmesan cheese
- ➢ ¼ cup of feta cheese crumbles
- ➢ ½ cup of shredded sharp cheddar cheese.

Preparation

1. First, it is important for you to slice the bacon to bite size. Fry the pieces over medium heat

while on a pan. This is let until the bacon is crunchy.

2. Once the bacon has become crispy, add the sliced cherry tomatoes then cook for about 4 minutes.
3. Whisk all the 10 eggs in a large bowl. Add the ¼-cup cream into the bowl then mix them appropriately.
4. Include the cheese in the bowl containing the whisked eggs-cream mixture. Use a spatula to make a homogeneous mixture.
5. The ultimate egg mixture is poured in a pan then allowed to cook for like 2 minutes.
6. Into an oven with a temperature of about 375 degrees Celsius, place the pan containing the egg mixture for about 25 minutes.
7. The meal is ready to serve 8 dishes.

Cooking the bacon appropriately will remove nitrates naturally present in it.

Broccoli with Lemon Butter

For fat fast recipes, this broccoli with lemon butter is one of the best meals to consider.

Knowing how to prepare them is, therefore, important to be sure you are not consuming the additives that might expose you to the other health issues.

Ingredients

> ➢ 2 tablespoon of butter
> ➢ ¼ fresh or frozen broccoli. This should be pound
> ➢ ¼ lemon

Recipe preparation

1. Considering your taste, steam the broccoli
2. Over the broccoli, melt the butter. Squeeze the lemon on the resultant mixture.
3. At a glance of an eye, the recipe is ready to kick off your day and putting your body in ketosis.

Sea Salt Cheese Crackers Gluten Free

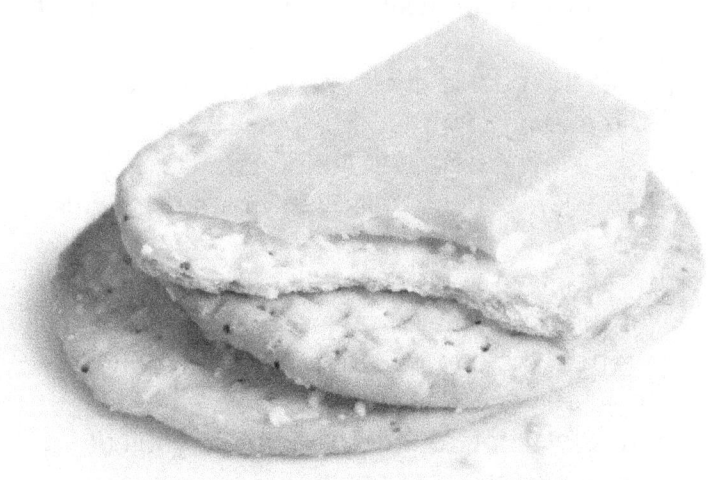

This meal is ideal for the lovers of crunchy foods. This meal has naturally satisfying characteristics and with no gluten. This meal can last for a long time when stored in the freezer.

Ingredients

➢ 1 cup of almond flour
➢ 1 egg
➢ ¼ cup of golden flax seed meal

- ½ teaspoon of baking soda
- ½ teaspoon of salt
- Salt
- 1 cup of sharp cheddar cheese
- 1½ tablespoon of sea salt

Recipe preparation

1. In a food processor, add the almond flour, salt, baking soda, flax seed, and cheese. Turn on the processor to ensure the ingredients combine homogeneously.
2. To the uniform mixture, add oil and egg to form a ball.
3. Onto the cookie sheet, press the formed balls to make a dough
4. Sprinkle the salt over the dough. Using your hands spread the salt evenly over the whole area.
5. Use a pizza cutter to cut the flat almond mixture into smaller shapes of your choice.
6. Preheat the oven to about 350F for about 15 minutes.
7. While still hot, retrace the shapes you cut earlier using a pizza cutter.
8. Allow 10 minutes to cool the meal before enjoying the service.

Simple Egg Salad w/Salmon

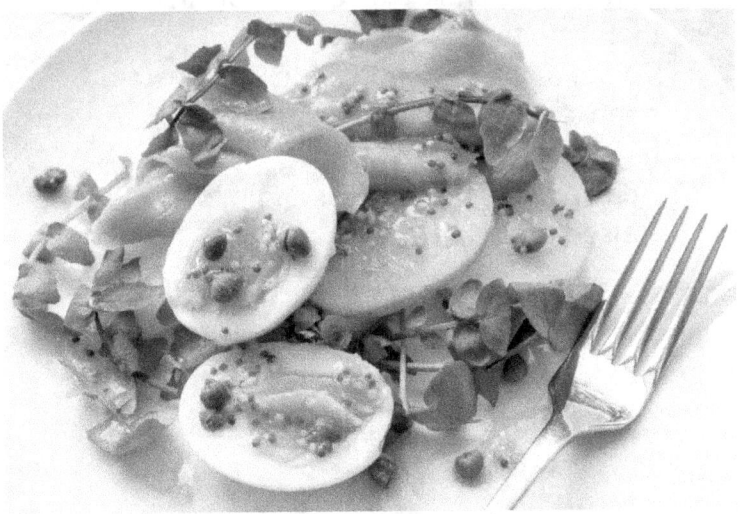

This is one of the best ketogenic recipes that lovers of eggs should enjoy its benefit. The fat contained in the eggs will help in the production of the ketone for energy supply to the brain cells.

This recipe is easy to prepare and requires a couple of spices to produce a nice flavor.

Ingredients

- ➢ 9 hardboiled eggs
- ➢ Salmon(optional)
- ➢ 2 tablespoon of mayo
- ➢ 1 stalk of celery
- ➢ 1 tablespoon of Dijon mustard
- ➢ ½ teaspoon of dill
- ➢ ¼ teaspoon of paprika
- ➢ Salt

Recipe preparation

1. Chop all the 9 hard-boiled eggs into a large bowl. Again chop the celery stalk then add them into the same bowl.
2. To the same bowl add the Dijon mustard, paprika, dill and the mayo then stir them together.
3. Add salt to taste then stir again to mix them well before enjoying the meal.

Not forgetting the lovers of the bacon, adding a couple of crispy strips for flavor will be an added advantage.

Mayo can also be substituted with the whole milk yogurt.

Scrumptious Tuna Salad

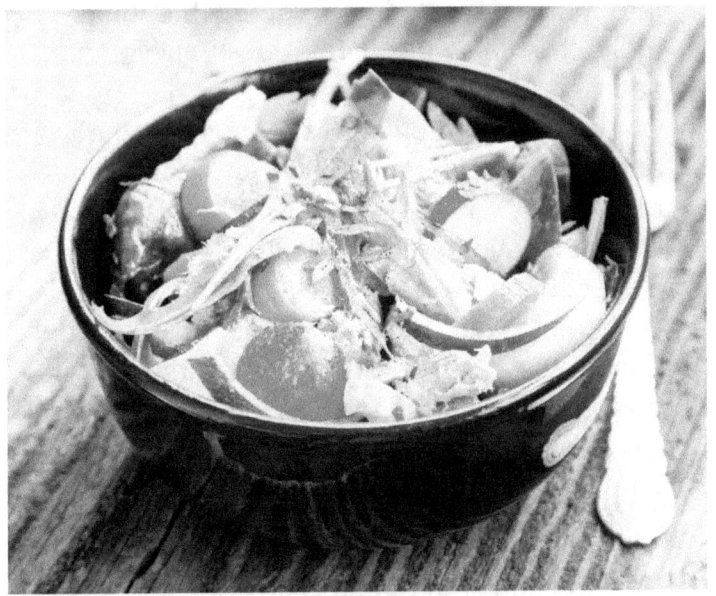

Fish is an example of white meat recommended by the physicians. The presence of the Omega-3 fatty acids in the tuna makes it ideal for those under ketosis.

A delicious snack or sometimes lunch can be made by following a simple recipe.

Ingredients

- 1 stalk of celery
- ½ cup of diced apples
- Two 5 Oz cans of Tuna
- 3½ tablespoon of mayo
- Juice from a half lemon
- ¼ cup of chopped roasted almonds
- ½ cup of diced red onion

Recipe preparation

1. Into a medium sized bowl, empty the tuna.
2. Flake the tuna while in the bowl until you are satisfied with the texture.
3. Chop the celery, onions, almonds and the apples then add them to the bowl containing the tuna.
4. Use the mayo to top the mixture.
5. Squeeze the half lemon to sprinkle the juice onto the mixture. (Before squeezing the lemon, ensure you remove all the seeds first).
6. Continue mixing the mixture together then add the pepper and salt for taste.
7. The meal is now ready to be served. Enjoy your meal.

The half lemon should be fresh. The cook should be careful to prevent the seeds from getting into the meal.

This salad can be enjoyed in a coconut pancake or even the lettuce wrap.

Hard Boiled Egg

Eggs are versatile either as a snack or as an ingredient in a salad. They are normally used for breakfast. This type of recipe ensures that the yolk does not overcook.

This diet is preferred for ketosis. Simple steps are involved in the preparation of this meal.

Ingredients

- ➢ 12 eggs

- ➢ ½ teaspoon of salt

Preparation instruction

1. The first step is arranging the eggs in a single layer in a saucepan.
2. Cover the eggs with about an inch of water.
3. To the water, add the salt into the water
4. Over a regulated heat, allow the eggs to boil.
5. Once the eggs begin to boil, remove the heat source for few seconds, then reduce the heat to low.
6. Over the reduced heat, allow the eggs to simmer for like a minute.
7. After the minute, let the eggs cool for like 12 minutes.
8. Use a slotted spoon to place the eggs in a bowl containing ice water. This helps in stopping the cooking process.
9. Enjoy the hard eggs

Pan Fried Crunchy Cheese Sticks

Cheese is one of the most popular high-fat low carb snack. This food can last for days when stored well in a refrigerator.

Ingredients

- ➢ 2 cups of sharp cheddar cheese
- ➢ 11/2 cup of parmesan cheese

Recipe preparation

1. Over a preheated pan, spread the cheese evenly.

2. Allow to cook until the cheese begin to turn brown.
3. Roll the cheese and enjoy your meal. This meal is enough for 3 serves.

For those who do not like the cheddar cheese, use any cheese of your own choice. This meal increases the fat content within the body enhancing ketosis.

5 Minute No Cook Lunch Salad

Taking a salad using the correct healthy ingredients ensure that one remains full until the next main meal. As indicated in the name, this diet does not require any source of heat since they don't need to cook. In about five minutes, this meal is ready for consumption.

Ingredients

- 1 red bell pepper
- 1 can tuna
- 1 heart of romaine
- 3 tablespoon of olive oil
- ¼ cup of cheese. For example the feta cheese
- Pepper
- Salt

Recipe preparation

1. After washing the romaine, tear the heart of romaine.
2. Add all the available ingredients in one medium size bowl then mix them together.
3. This salad is now ready for consumption.

The pepper and the salt are to add taste to your salad.

This salad meal is enough for 2 serves.

Grass Fed Steak

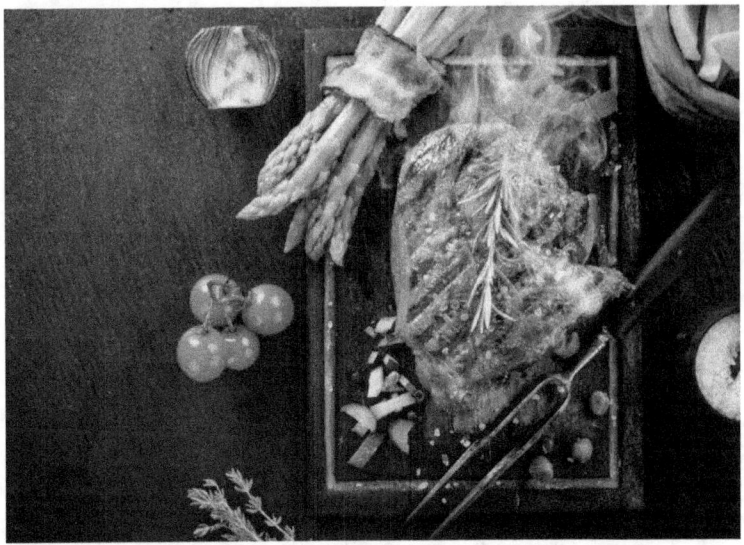

The grass fed steak contain less fat compared to the grain fed ones. This meal, therefore, requires a gentle cooking procedure.

Before cooking the steak from a freezer, let it for about an hour. This brings it to room temperature. Sprinkle pepper and salt evenly over the raw meat.

Ingredients

- ➢ Any piece of steak
- ➢ 2 tablespoon of grass fed butter
- ➢ Pepper
- ➢ Salt

Recipe preparation

1. Remove the steak from the freezer an hour before cooking it. This ensures that the food achieves the room temperature.
2. After the hour, generously cover the steak with both the pepper and salt.
3. For about 200F, preheat the oven before heating up an ovenproof skillet over medium to high heat.
4. Sear the steak for about 2 minutes.
5. Depending on the thickness of the steak, cook for about 10 to 20 minutes.
6. Allow the ready meal to cool for like 10 minutes then enjoy the ketogenic benefits of the meal.

In addition

When it comes to a keto diet, choosing the good fat is vital. The bad fat will come with other side effects like the elevating cholesterol level. Considering the many simple ketogenic recipes has proven to be a good strategy for maintaining our body in ketosis for its several outstanding health benefits.

CHAPTER EIGHT: Ketogenic Diet Desserts

Desserts are the meal course that is consumed after the main meal. To many, having this end meal after the normal meal makes them feel good. This dish is seen as an unhealthy eating practice. On the positive side of this context, desserts have proven to have many health benefits.

The desire to consume the dessert comes when the insulin level shoots to an abnormal level forcing an emergency intake of carbohydrates. This rise in the insulin level can be after a heavy meal done at irregular intervals.

The triggered insulin production will lead to decreased blood glucose level hence craving for the sweet foods after the meal. Elimination of high-carb foods can also make one desire the tasty after meal course.

This becomes a concern when it comes to those under ketogenic diet. It states that the uncontrolled intake of sweet foods will cause adverse effects to your health. The ketogenic principle says that we should cut the starch and replace them with fat.

When it comes to dessert, dieticians have researched on several foods that can be taken as an after meal to make you feel good. It is, therefore, important for those under this condition to know how to prepare the dessert to sustain their feelings.

Some of the common dessert recipes that are of great help

Most of the dessert recipes are easy to prepare to top up the main course. Some of them are illustrated in this chapter to meet the dream of lovers of the dessert while trying to maintain ketosis within the body.

1) Keto Strawberry Shortcake Dessert Recipe

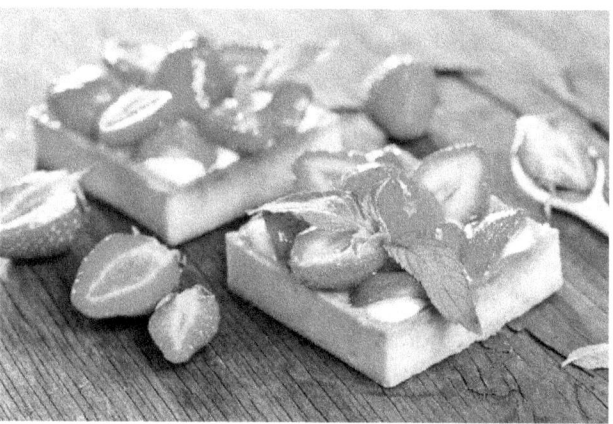

This is recipe takes less time to be ready. This dessert is taken while cold hence the need to have a refrigerator or an improvised cooling system.

Ingredients

- ½ tablespoon of butter
- 2 tablespoon of almond meal
- 1 cup of chopped strawberries
- 1 teaspoon of sugar-free vanilla syrup (for those who prefer sweeteners)
- ½-cup cream

Recipe preparation

1. Add the butter, and the almond meal to a mug then place it in the oven for about 8-10 minutes. Preheat oven to 375 degrees F (190 C).

2. Use the spoon bottom to flatten the mixture and form a flat crust-like substance

3. Add the chopped blackberries into the mug containing the almond butter crust.

4. Blend the ½-cup heavy cream in a blender. This is the stage where you can add the sugar-free vanilla syrup as a sweetener.

5. Add the blended cream containing a sweetener (not a must) into the cup with the butter-almond meal combination.

6. For the crust to cool and be bread-like, place the mixture in the refrigerator for about 30 minutes.

7. After the timed a half an hour, the dessert is ready to be consumed as an after meal to meet your body desires.

2) Keto Lemon Custard Tarts with Almond Lavender Crust

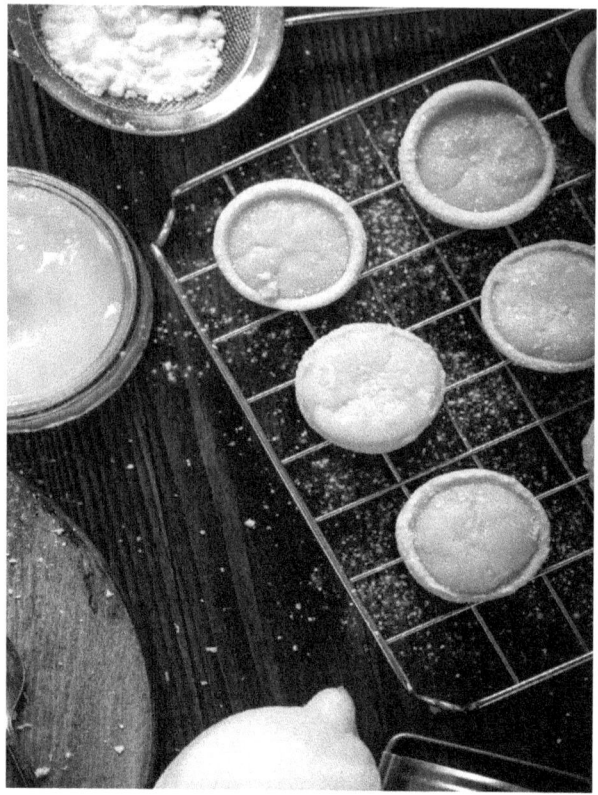

This dessert must be left overnight to chill before it is ready for use. The recipe is favorable to the lovers of the lavender. If you do not like it, then this dessert is not recommended to you.

Ingredients

Preparation of the filling and the crust are done separately using different ingredients.

For crust

➢ ¾ cup of almond meal
➢ ½ tablespoon of dried lavender flowers
➢ 3 tablespoon of unsalted butter
➢ 1 tablespoon of sugar-free vanilla syrup

For the fillings

➢ 4 egg yolks
➢ ½ cup of squeezed lemon juice
➢ Grated zest of 3 lemons
➢ ½ cup of unsalted butter
➢ ½ cup of sugar-free vanilla syrup

Preparation procedures

1.   To about 375 degrees Celsius, preheat the oven.

2.   Grease two crème Brulee dishes (the two plate are for two serves)

3.   Using a mortar and pestle, grind the lavender flower to fine texture

4.   Melt the butter and mix it with lavender and almond flour. Press this mixture into the bottom of the dishes

5.   Bake, the mixture until the top, begins to turn brown. This can take up to 10 minutes. This is now the crust. The set is aside for some time.

6.   Begin making the fillings by blending the 4 egg yolks mixed with lemon juice, lavender, lemon zest and ½ cup of melted butter. This is done until the mixture becomes homogenous.

7.   Transfer the filling to a saucepan to cook at medium to low temperatures. This is allowed to cook for about 15 minutes, and in the process, constant stirring will allow a thick padding.

8.   Empty the filling on the lavender-almond crust in both the dishes

9.   Use plastic wraps to cover the dishes then put the dishes in a freezer overnight before the dessert is ready for consumption.

10.   The following day, the recipe is ready for a dessert.

For those who do not like the lavender, the recipe can still be great without the sweetener. Try it and enjoy the benefit of this keto dessert.

3) Instant avocado vanilla pudding (vegan)

This simple and velvety dessert is recommended for the vegetarians who do not like any dairy product. This instant preparation will be convenient in case of a dessert emergency.

Ingredients

- ➢ 1 can of organic coconut milk
- ➢ 80 drops of liquid stevia
- ➢ 2 teaspoons organic vanilla extract
- ➢ 2 ripe avocado. Peeled and sliced into chunks
- ➢ 1 tablespoon of freshly squeezed lime juice.

Recipe preparation

1. Into a blender, add all the ingredients then blend them until they become smooth. This is done while the lid is covered.

The nutritious value of this dessert cannot be underestimated. Best for the non-meat eaters.

4) Watermelon Cream Soup

This is one of the important desserts that its value is underestimated. This takes a maximum of 10 minutes to be ready.

Ingredients

> 2 tablespoons of organic sour cream
> ¾ seeded watermelon chunks
> ¼ cup of raspberries
> ¼ teaspoon of freshly squeezed lemon juice
> 1 tablespoon of sugar-free vanilla
> ¼ teaspoon of chopped mint. Should be fresh
> ½ cup of freshly whipped cream

Recipe preparation

1. Into the blender, add the raspberries, watermelon, sour cream lemon juice, chopped mints and the sugar-free vanilla as the sweetener. Blend them until they become smooth

2. Empty the ready soup in a bowl then top with the whipped cream. This is served immediately.

The above desserts among other important ones are keto-friendly and should be added as a ketogenic remedy for adverse health effects. They are also sweet to meet your desire without adding extra glucose that would interfere with ketosis.

Supplementation for the ketogenic dieting

This innovation was aimed at making the individuals lose weight by shedding off the extra fat within their body. Maintaining the muscle tone is important during this trying moment. With keto diet, this can be made possible by including some supplements to the diet.

1. Regular intake of water

When subjecting yourself to this type of intervention in order to cut weight, it is important to take large amounts of water. About two gallons of water will do in ensuring the correct muscle mass. This is because, during this process, the water level also drops and therefore should be topped up.

2. Creatine

For a good body shape, creatine level has to be elevated forcing the muscle tissues to hold an additional amount of water. This helps in maintaining a bigger muscle tone when under this therapeutic procedure.

Before embarking on the ketogenic dieting, visit your physician for a complete blood panel. This will help you have knowledge on the careful use of the available supplements. This innovation possesses stress to the body. This is the reason as to why you should consider using the supplements.

CHAPTER Nine: More Food Ideas with Images

In this chapter I will provide you more ideas about low-carb and Ketogenic meals and snacks that are essential to have for two reasons that I can think of:

1-You need a variety of foods to save yourself from the boredom of having the same food day in and day out. That way you can stay on Ketogenic or low-carb diet much longer and achieve your goal whether it is weight loss or for other health reasons. This is very important for children so they can enjoy various tastes, colors, and textures of foods.

2-The second reason has to do with consuming different micronutrients such as vitamins, minerals, phytochemicals, enzymes, and the list goes on.

You will not see recipes per say but mostly self-explanatory images and with few words of explanation to guide you in the right direction. I have chosen the below list randomly out of my own experience, but as they say, the sky is the limit so don't be concerned with trying new foods to spice up your life a little bit more.

Here we go:

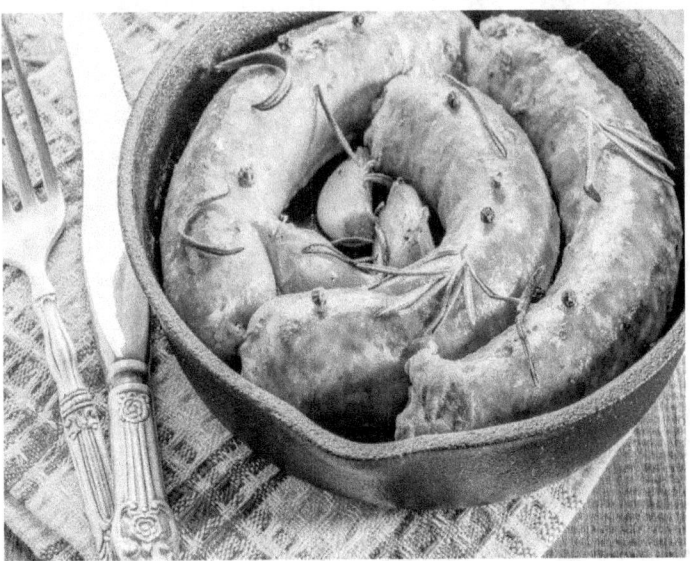

Figure 1 Rustic style fried sausages

This rustic looking sausage can add a nice spicy flavor and qualifies for Keto or Low-carb meals since the fat content is high. The sausage can be cooked in different ways such as sautéed, grilled, or lightly fried. Make sure to look for the best quality that you can find without any artificial flavors or preservatives. Or even better you can make them yourself.

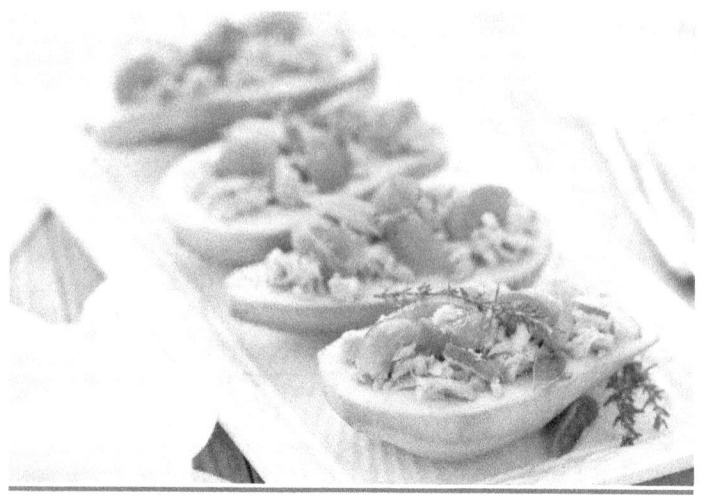

Figure 2 Avocado, tuna and tomato salad

Avocados can be eaten in many different ways and here is another idea to enjoy your fat, protein, and some carbs.

Depending on what diet you are following but since the ketogenic diet is more limited than low-carb diet regarding protein amount and of course carbohydrates. So you need to watch your protein intake and in this case is limit your consumption of tuna due to its high content of protein.

The same thing goes for tomatoes since they are relatively high in carbs if you compare them to other leafy vegetables.

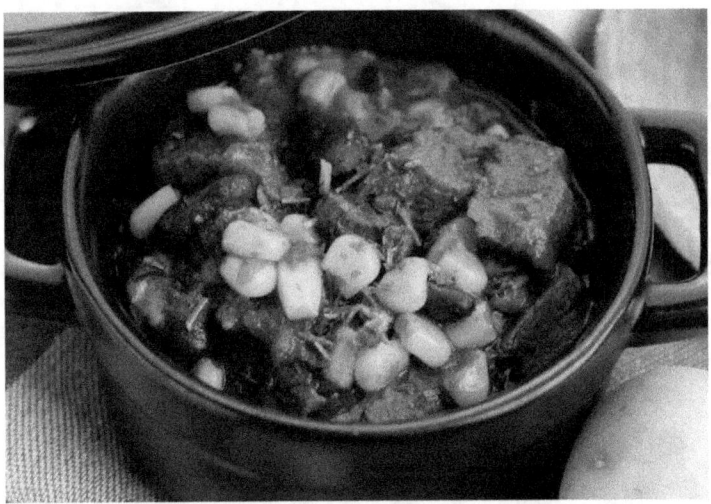

Figure 3 Delicious winter traditional hot pot stew with meat and vegetables

This tasty meat and vegetable stew will give you satiety due to its nutrient dense profile and not to mention the taste is just wonderful. This meal has been traditionally prepared during the winter season, but it is up to you to have whenever you wish.

Again this meal is high in protein, so you need to be conscious of it. Including a few beans and corn is fine and you can be more liberal with the amount if you are following the low-carb diet.

Now if you are following the Keto-diet you want to increase the fat content and decrease the protein and carbohydrate contents. How do I go about that, you might ask?

Well this is what I suggest:

-Add more butter

-Add some olive oil

-Add some of the coconut oil

-Add some sour cream

-Include some of the creamy cheese such as Brie

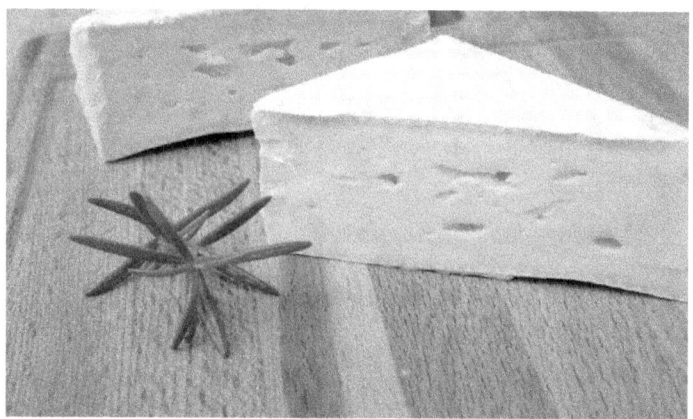

Figure 4 Brie Cheese

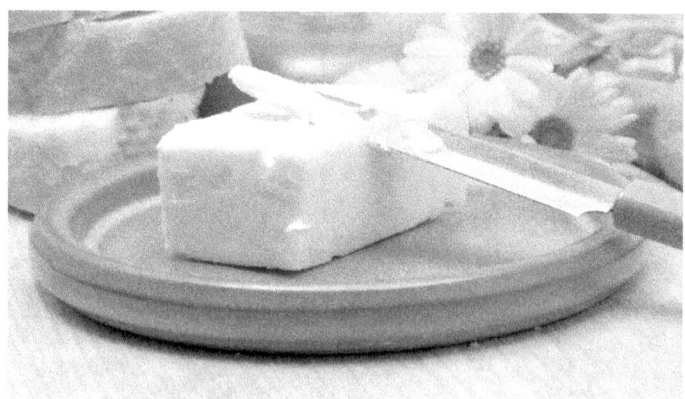

Figure 5 Grass Fed Butter

To me, Brie cheese and butter are almost a mandatory food items in my diet whether it is Ketogenic or not. They contain fat-soluble vitamins such as A, K, and D. Not to mention they are very satisfying and versatile in combining them with other foods and butter in particular.

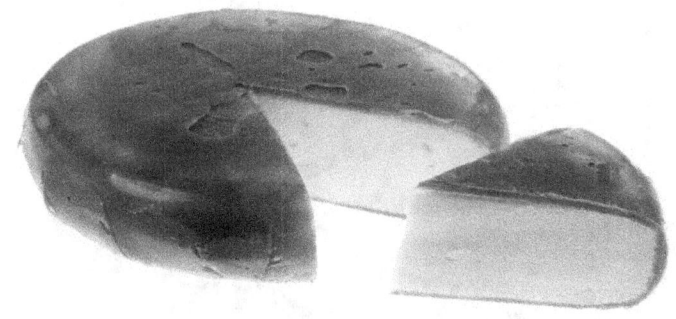

Figure 6 Dutch Edam Gouda cheese

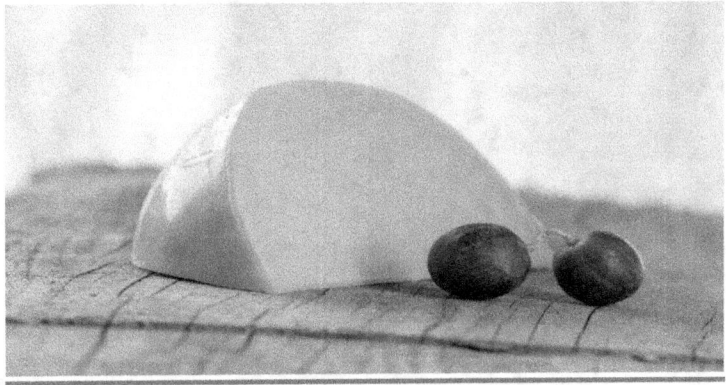

Figure 7 Hollander Cheese

Gouda and Hollander have aged cheeses and with aged cheese, the content of lactose that is a milk sugar becomes less and less due to the fermentation process. Therefore, these cheeses are Ketogenic and low-carb friendly.

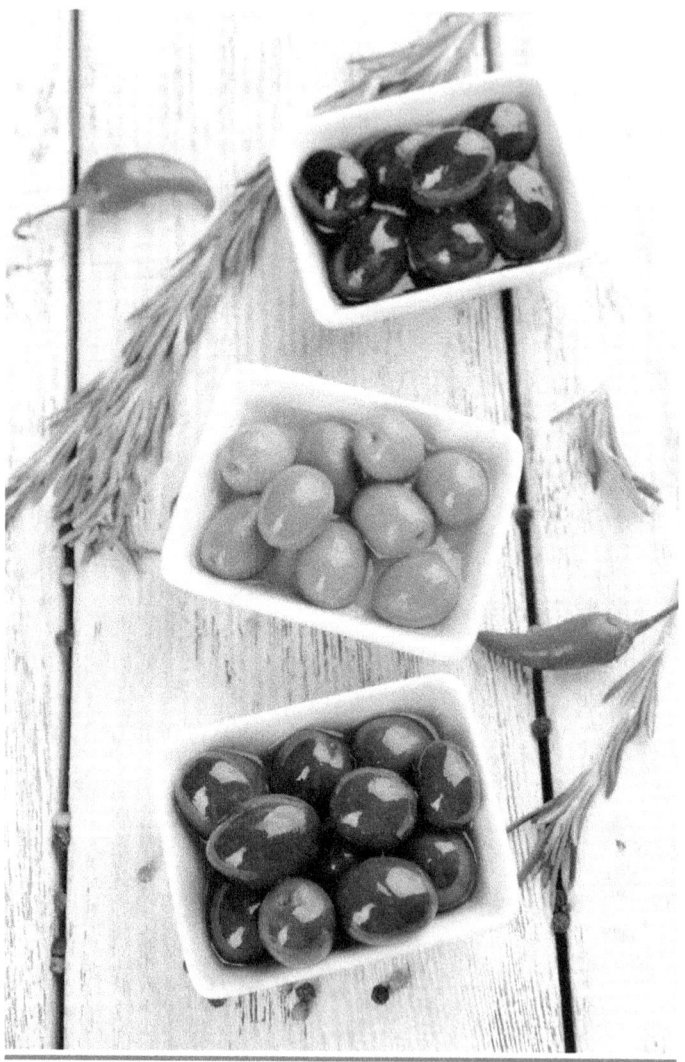

Figure 8 Different marinated olives

Olives make good condiments as part of a snack or a meal. They are relatively low in carbs and high in fat.

Not only that but they are loaded with antioxidants and other phytochemicals. I recommend using olives preserved in natural brine and stored in a glass jar.

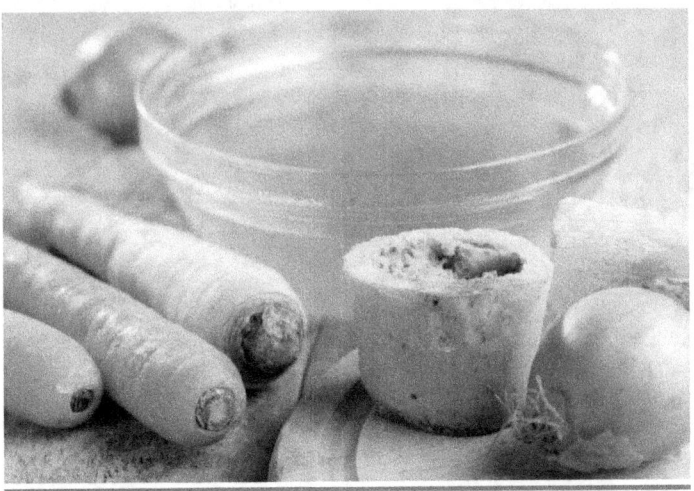

Figure 9 Bowl of beef broth

What not to like about bone broth! Bone broth is a traditional meal that has been used for thousands of years. It is basically cooking bone in water with some vinegar and adding few leafy vegetables if you like and some pepper and salt.

Here is a book I recommend that is short read and to point which talks about bone broth and Meat stock by Ben Alexi

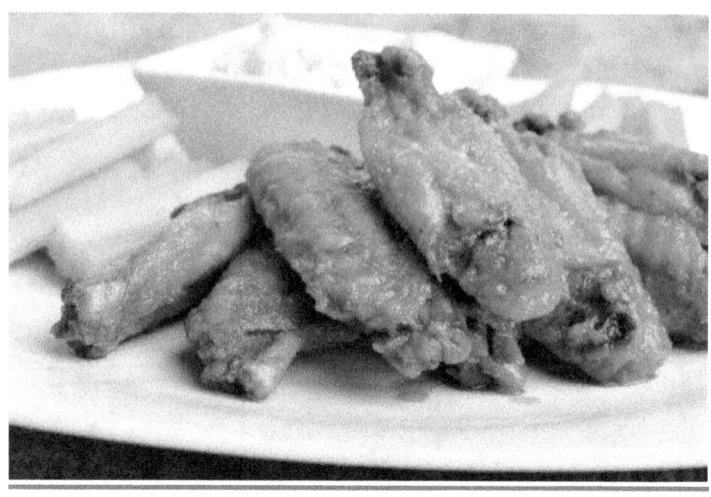

Figure 10 Chicken wings

A meal like spicy chicken wings and using sour cream to cool it off just a bit and low carb vegetable such as celery are a tasty ketogenic meal.

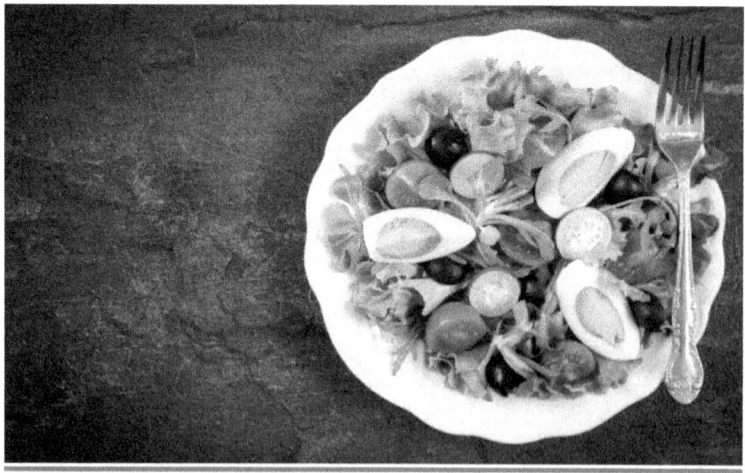

Figure 11 Boiled eggs salad

Boiled eggs can be included in many meals, and a salad is one of the best choices.

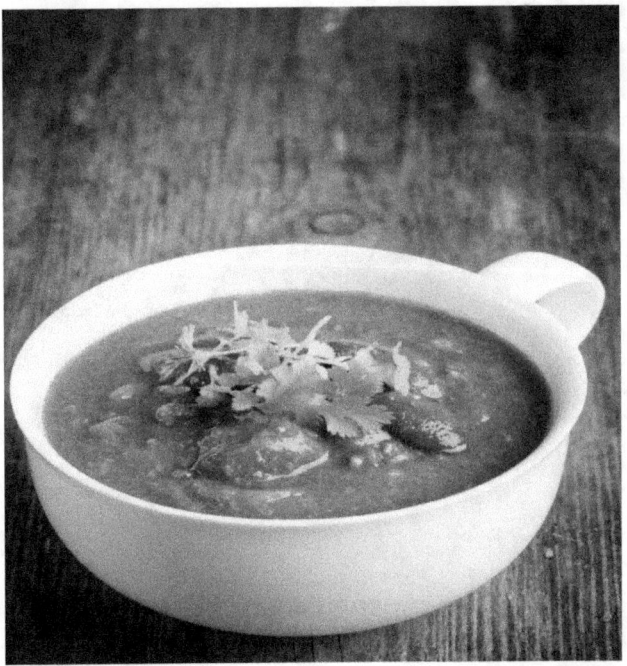

Figure 12 Chili

Before you make chili purchase ground beef that is 80% or 85% lean meat. Any leaner than that then you risk consuming more protein in your chili meal. And leaner meat tastes too dry and doesn't provide satiety as much as the high fat content meat.

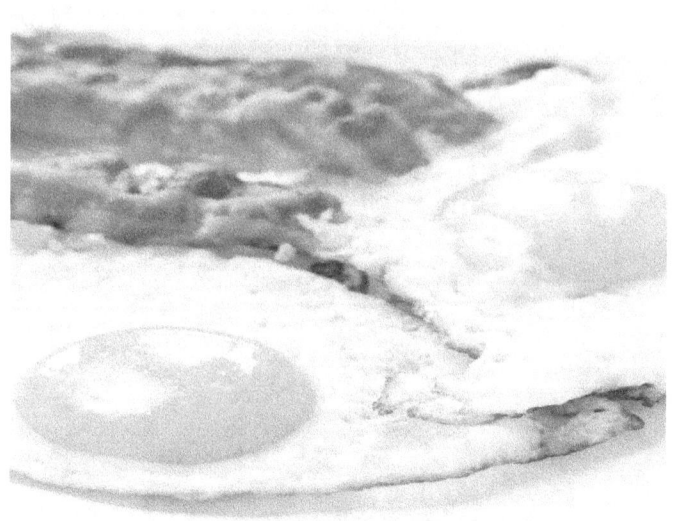

Figure 13 Eggs and bacon

One of the best meals you can have for breakfast is bacon and eggs regarding taste and keeping you satisfied for several hours to come.

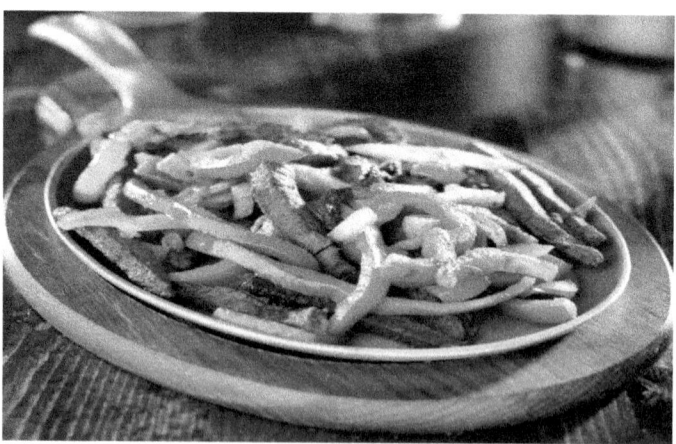

Figure 14 Beef fajitas and bell peppers

If you make fajitas yourself, try to choose a meat cut with fat in it and not too lean. You can include several slices of bell peppers and tomatoes as well to keep the most balanced.

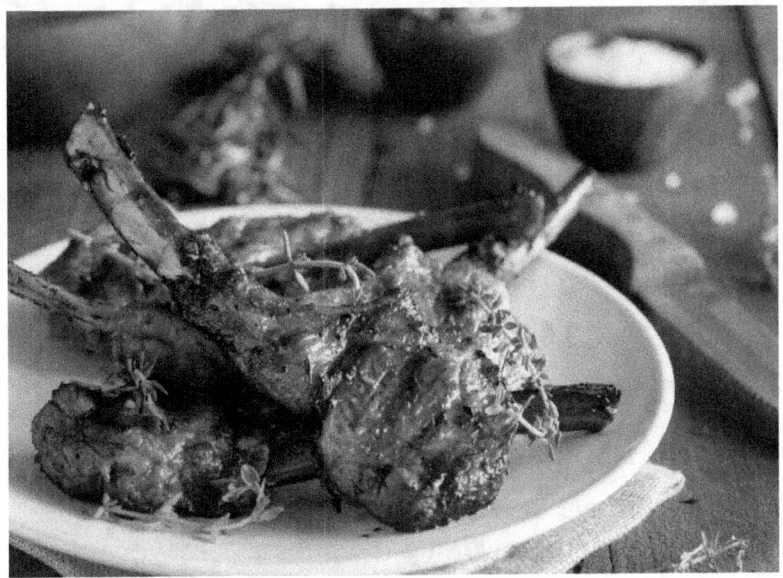

Figure 15 Grilled Lamb Chops

In general, lamb meat has a higher amount of fat than beef and lamb chops are among the best meat part of a lamb, and it is succulent and very satisfying.

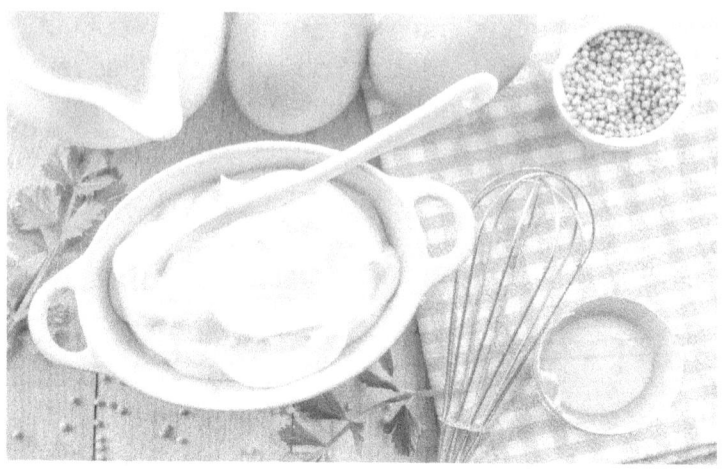

Figure 16 Mayonnaise

Homemade mayonnaise is your best option can choose good quality of oil such as olive or avocado oil. It is also affordable in the long run. However, if you don't have the time here are two brands that I have used and provided good quality of mayonnaise:

-Wilderness Family Naturals and - Primal Kitchen Avocado Oil Mayo

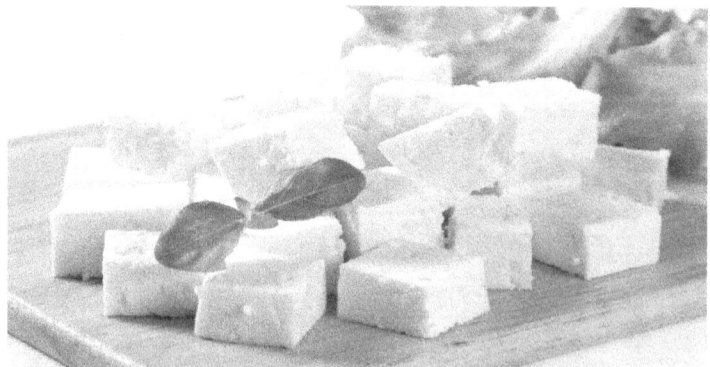

Figure 17 Feta cheese

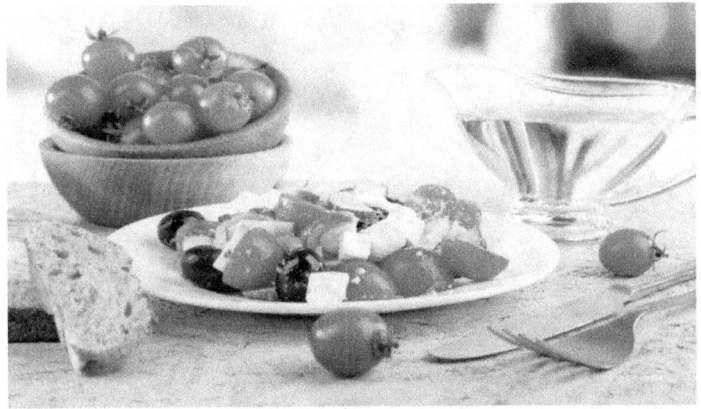

Figure 18 Greek Salad Feta Cheese

Feta cheese is another good source of fat, protein, and low in carbs. Having a Greek Salad Feta cheese is very refreshing in hot summer weather and don't forget to drizzle over it some extra virgin olive oil!

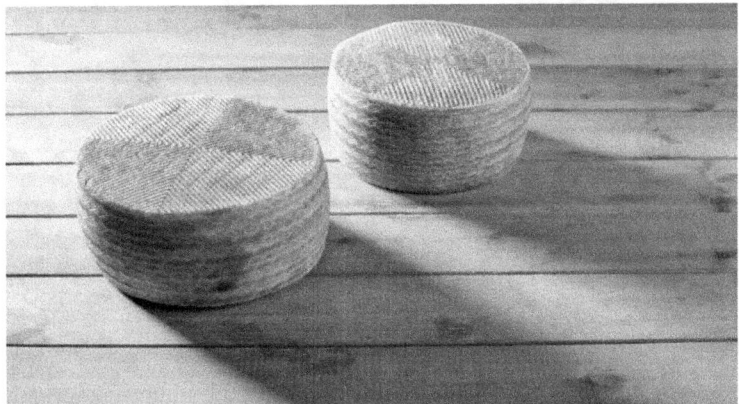

Figure 19 Manchego aged cheese

Excellent choice of cheese! Manchego is Spanish cheese that has been aged for several months, so the carbohydrates content is even lower than other less aged cheeses.

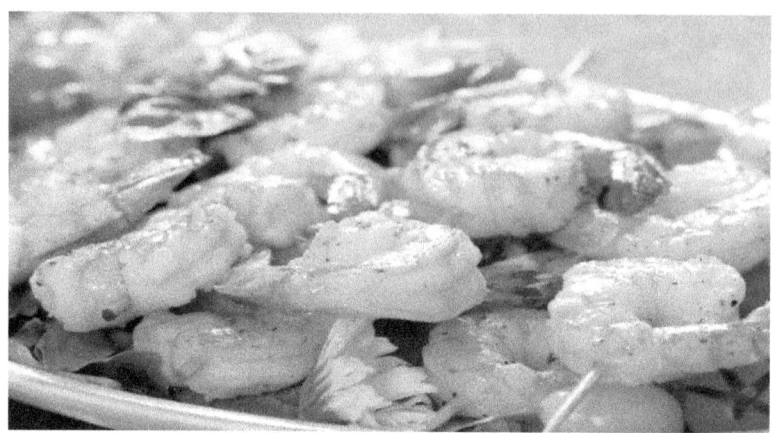

Figure 20 Shrimp skewered

Shrimp is a rich source of fat-soluble vitamins, and some researchers estimate that wild shrimp has eight to ten times of vitamin D than nutrient dense animal products such as organ meats! Shrimp is low in fat and high in protein so that I would melt some butter or olive oil or even both.

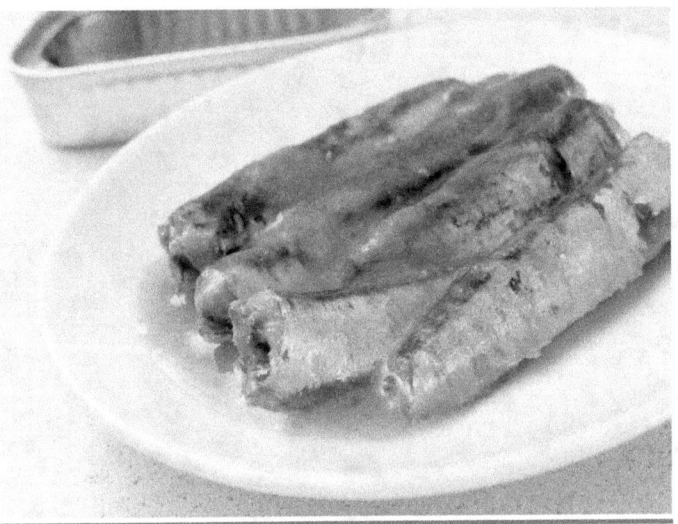

Figure 21 Sardines

Sardines like anchovies are an excellent source of calcium and various minerals. At the same time, they are rich in and B12 and fat-soluble vitamins A and D.

Do your best in choosing sardines that are not deboned nor skinless whenever possible. Sardines are usually packed in water or some type of vegetable oil. I suggest you choose sardines packed in water or olive oil which are the best.

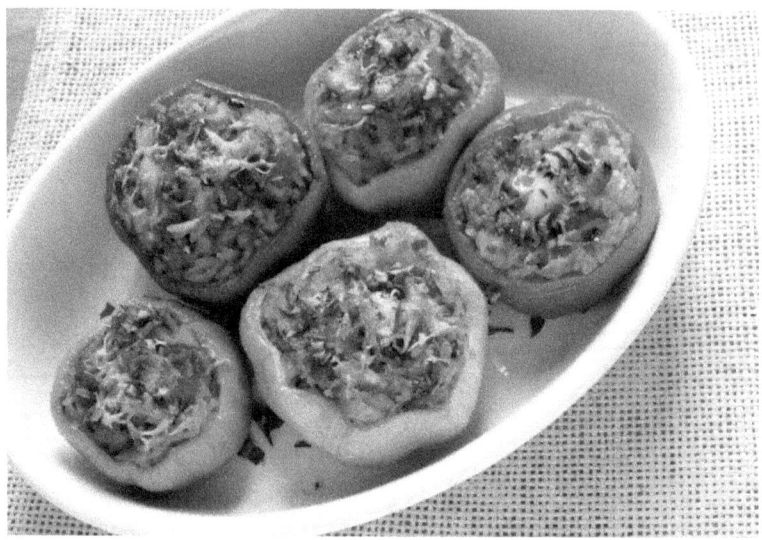

Figure 22 Stuffed peppers

Stuffed peppers are very delicious however to enjoy a low-carb or Ketogenic stuffed peppers you are most likely to be out of luck since most prepared ones are high in carbs such as rice.

It is relatively easy to make so replace the rice with your favorite ground meat and mixed with a few grated carrots or oatmeal. That way the meat is moisture and tender.

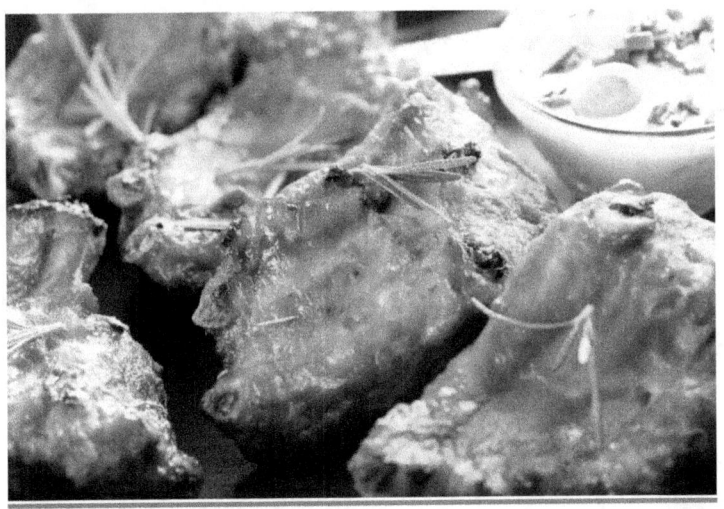

Figure 23 Spare ribs with sour cream

There is nothing much to say about spare ribs with sour cream except enjoy this mouthwatering low-carb meal!

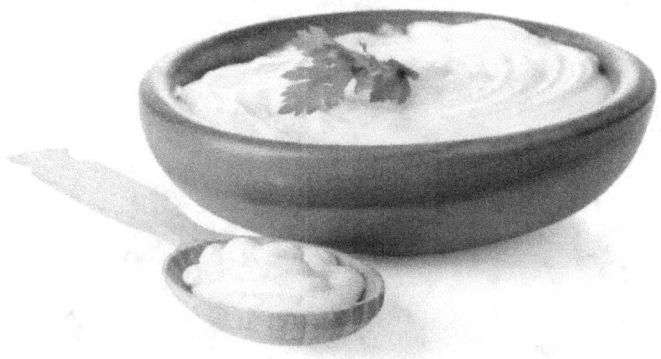

Figure 24 Sour cream

Enjoy sour cream with few carrot or celery sticks for a nice afternoon snack.

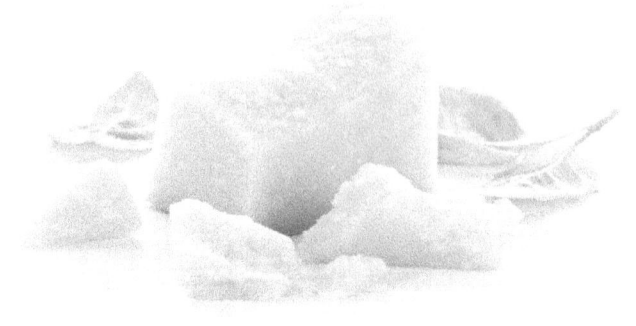

Figure 25 Parmesan cheese

Parmesan cheese such as the Italian Parmigiano-Reggiano kind is aged for at least for two years therefore the milk sugar content is very low and the taste is distinctive and divine.

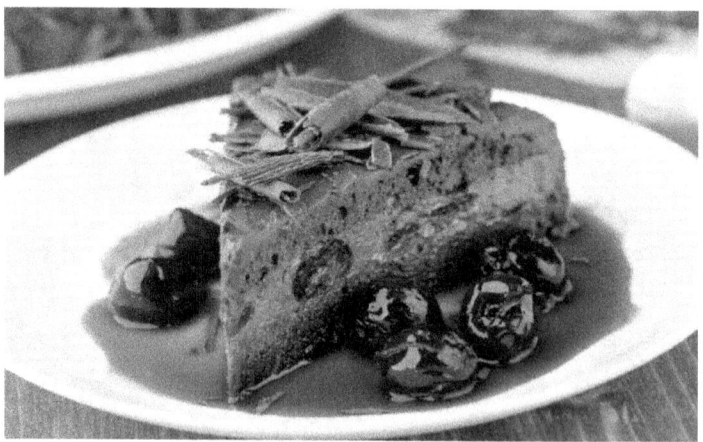

Figure 26 Chocolate mousse cake with dark cherries

More ideas for dessert and you just need to be extra careful with your ingredients since you need to replace them with more Ketogenic ingredients. The conventional recipe for Chocolate mousse cake calls for 7 ounces semi-sweet baking chocolate

- Butter
- Eggs
- Cream of tartar
- Stevia
- Egg yolks
- Vanilla extract
- Whipped cream
- Powdered sugar

All the above ingredients qualify for Ketogenic and low-carb dessert except the powdered sugar. However, in my experience using Stevia alone is not the best idea for enjoying sweets just because it tastes too sweet and has an after taste flavor that did not agree with me very well.

I would replace the powdered sugar with maple syrup which still has sugar in it. But make between the stevia and maple syrup you will have a balanced amount of sugar.

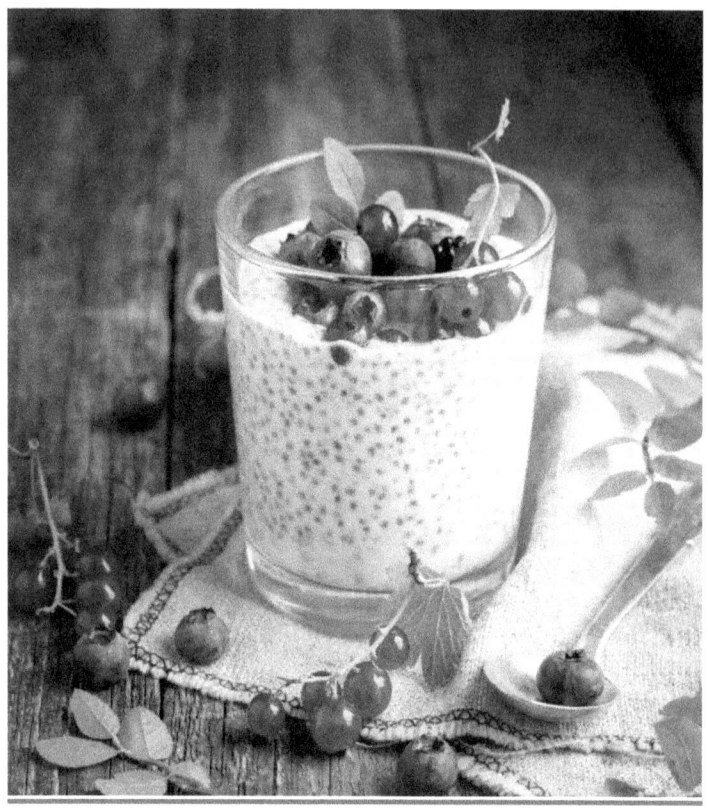

Figure 27 Yogurt with chia seeds and fresh berries

Yogurt is relatively low in sugar than whole milk, and that is due to the fermentation process occurs in yogurt but it still has some sugar in it, so you need to be careful there. Chia is a healthful seed, and it has about 5 grams of carbohydrates.

However, 3 of these grams are fibrous which has little effect on raising blood glucose. You can also add few full-of-antioxidant blueberries, raspberries, blackberries, or cherries.

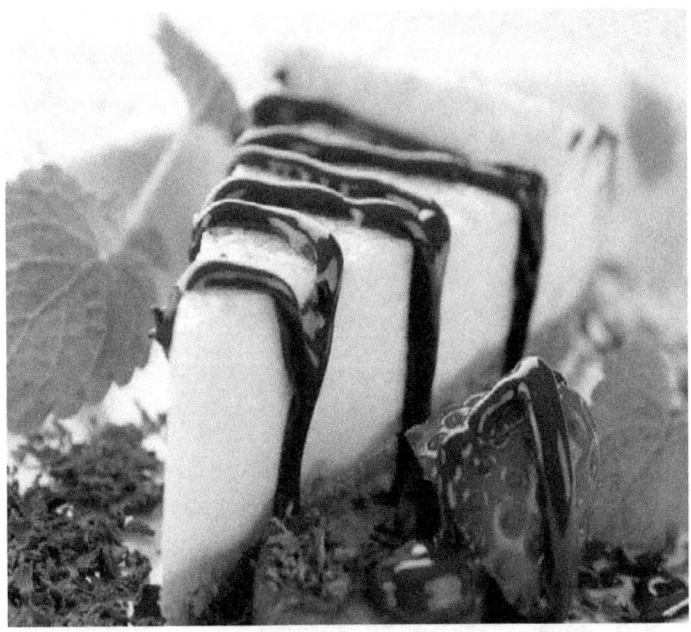

Figure 28 Cheesecake slice with chocolate

Cheesecake is made from cheese cream which is a low-carb food but here are few things you want to change:

-You can use a crustless cheesecake or a low-carb crust such as almond or other types of crushed nuts. You can mix the cream cheese with stevia or a mixed of other sweeteners mentioned in the previous chapter. Finally, you can top it with drizzled dark chocolate syrup to enjoy.

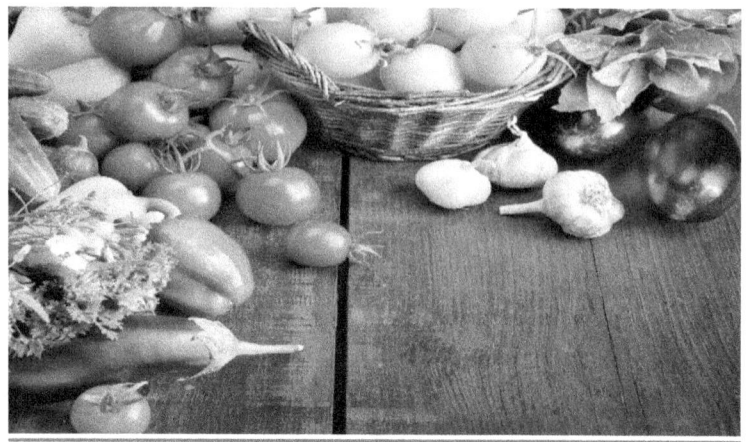

Figure 29 Less starchy vegetables

Use less starchy vegetables for your ketogenic meals and don't forget to include vegetables of different colors and tastes so you can ensure getting various nutrients from all kinds of vegetables.

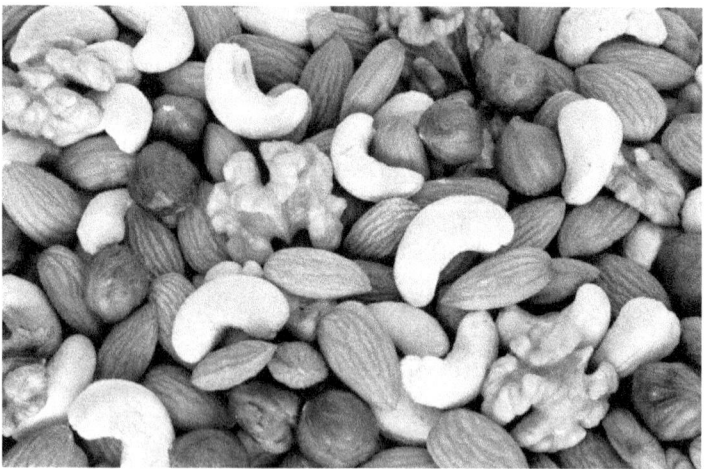

Figure 30 Mixed of raw nuts: almonds, filberts, walnuts, and cashews

Nuts are very nutrient dense, delicious snack or combined with a small meal. They are high in fat and moderate in carbs and particular cashews. So enjoy them however in a limited amount.

CHAPTER Ten: Important Ketogenic Diet FAQ

Supplements on Keto Diet

According to scientists, the ketogenic diet is effective in harmonizing the body system. Regardless of the health benefits of this diet, switching to the ketogenic diet is not an easy task. Supplements, therefore, help the body adapt to this new system.

An example of a supplement that allows the body to perform well in a low-carb diet with high-fat concentration is sodium. When in ketogenic diet, sodium, and water are excreted very fast. This lowers the blood sugar level due to the drop in the blood pressure. Symptoms of this are like the lightheadedness and sluggishness.

Adding about 1 gram of sodium after every 30 minutes before your daily workout will help the body adapt well when under ketogenic diet.

Other than the ketogenic supplements, there are some of the concerns that arise from keto diet that ought to be addressed professionally. Some of the questions frequently asked to include the following:

1. What you need to know about Ketosis vs. Ketoacidosis

These two terms normally confuse and hence the need for clarification. Ketosis, as described earlier in the book, means the state in which the body uses ketone bodies as the primary source of energy. The brain cells among other body cells use the energy supply from the ketones to function normally. Ketones are produced when the body system utilizes the fat consumed at the expense of the carbs. This is possible when the individual is under a ketogenic diet where he or she consumes meals that are high in fat concentration and low in carbs.

Ketoacidosis, on the other hand, is a health condition that is characterized by the acidification of blood. This results from the elevated levels of ketones or the sugar within the blood. This is usually a complication affecting those suffering from type 1 diabetes. This condition is deadly if not managed early.

2. Ketogenic diet and Glucophage

Glucophage is a glucose disposal agent that helps in dropping the sugar level and as a result, induce ketosis. The drug will heighten the sensitivity of the body to insulin. Glucophage is ingested together with the carb meals but forces the sugar to move to the muscle tissues and let the fat be metabolized to produce the required energy. This important drug also suppresses the appetite as well as reducing hunger in between the meals.

Though this drug is of great help in maintaining our body in ketosis, it has some side effects that should as well be managed: breathing problems, muscle pain, and weakness and feeling dizzy among others.

3. Ketogenic diet and Creatine supplements

For muscle contraction, energy is required. Individuals under this diet need to supplement their diet with this drug to help in re-phosphorylate the ADP to ATP that fuels the muscle actions. The water retention property of this drug is also important minimizing excessive water loss by the body.

Considering the side effects, several types of research say confirms that the correct usage of this supplement has no adverse effects.

4. Are Ketogenic and Low-carb diets for everyone?

Ketogenic and low-carb diet are helpful to many individuals but probably not everyone. However, it is important we consult our medical practitioners before we embark on a keto diet. For example, those who are naturally thin require close monitoring during this period of ketosis. Additional fat calories have to be added. There are many people who need a higher amount of carbohydrates to function well on a daily basis, so the question is what type of carbs? I would think these individuals need whole foods carbs such as fruits, vegetables, legumes, and whole grains that are prepared properly.

5. Hypothyroidism and Adrenal Fatigue!

Hypothyroid is a medical condition in which the thyroid gland fails to function normally since the inactive T4 hormone are not activated to the T3 hormone. Insulin is responsible for this action. Low-carb intake will mean low insulin count and hence hypothyroidism. In the case of this condition, jumping to moderate carbs intake will help in controlling this condition.

Adrenal fatigue, on the other hand, results from the very low intake of low-carb foods. This condition arises due to the dysregulation of the cortisol hormone due to adrenal stressors. If this is the case, up the intake of carbs to control the pressure.

6. What is Resistant Starch and How Helpful it is?

Resistant starch is sugar that reaches the colon undigested. This starch does not produce the needed energy within the body since the mouth, stomach, and the small intestines lack the enzymes capable of metabolizing prebiotics. This resistant starch appears in four different forms:

- RS type 1

This is usually found in grains, legumes, and the seeds. The starch has fibrous cell walls and is physically inaccessible to the digestive enzymes.

- RS type2

These foods with amylose are indigestible while still raw. Some examples of foods containing this resistant starch include the green bananas, potatoes, and the plantains. Cooking these foods causes changes to the amylose hence making the starch digestible and removing the resistant starch. Eating the cooked potatoes will interfere with ketosis process.

- RS type 3 (also known as the retrograde RS)

This prebiotic result when either the type 1 or type 2 resistant starch are cooked and cooled. Cooling the already cooked type 2 sources of foods will help regain the benefits of the resistant starch. Reheating the cooled foods for less than 130 degrees will not eliminate the resistant starch. An example includes the cooked and cooled potatoes as well as the cooked and cooled legumes.

- RS type 4.

This type of prebiotic is added as a supplement. An example is the Hi-maize resistant starch. The professional dietitians do not recommend this type 4 resistant starch.

The primary importance of the resistant starch is their ability to feed the useful bacteria found within the large intestine. This also helps in lowering the blood glucose level due to boosted insulin sensitivity.

7. Ketogenic diet and Cortisol Levels

In the case of exposure to stressors in our daily activities, our body usually fails to regulate the cortisol hormone. This will lead to certain disorder conditions like the adrenal fatigue.

The ketogenic diet, other than providing the energy fuel, will maintain a favorable blood sugar level elevating insulin sensitivity. This will, as a result, reduce the damaging effect of cortisol on the body.

8. A ketogenic diet as long-term, is it realistic and does it work?

Studies examine the short-term effects of ketogenic diets sidelining its long-term benefits. If possible, it is important to follow the keto diet until your life ends.

This diet has been important in reducing of extra weight as well as in the management of epilepsy and diabetes type 2 among other health benefits.

9. What is cyclical ketogenic diet?

This is a cyclic keto diet with intermittent high or moderate starch consumption to help the body adapt to the new body system under this diet. This also maximizes the fat loss.

10. Ketogenic diet side effects with Constipation

Many individuals complain about being constipated when they follow a ketogenic diet, and one good solution is to slightly increase the amount of salt or sea salt by about ½ teaspoon a day. When you begin the ketogenic diet physiologically, you will excrete more salt via the kidney, therefore, many individuals experience constipation.

CONCLUSION

The ketogenic diet involves the intake of foods rich in fat but with reduced amount of carbs. The fat becomes the primary source of energy instead of the usual sugar. This puts the body in ketosis: a state where they use the ketones produced from burning down the fats. The ketone bodies provide the desired energy to the brain cells and the other body cells.

The ketogenic diet is similar to the Atkins only that in keto diet, the lost carbs are replaced by consuming extra fat. This process has several health benefits. For example, ketosis helps our bodies lose extra weight. Management of other chronic conditions like epilepsy and diabetes has made this program an important health intervention even in the current generation.

Several foods are considered ketogenic due to their low-carb properties but rich in fat. These foods are combined into recipes that when consumed by the beneficiaries enhances ketosis. Ketogenic desserts are also available to facilitate the attainment of the ultimate goal of maintaining the body in ketosis to experience the resulting benefits.

Regular testing of the ketone concentration within the body is a healthy practice since it allows you to identify whether your body is out of balance. A home meter is available to help in giving the overview of your ketone properties. Visiting a professional to carry out this test is important to give you the exact state of your blood ketone composition.

Before beginning the ketogenic diet, it is important to consult your physician to detect any condition that might lead to complications. While in the diet, the physician is also mandated to monitor your progress to ensure your prime goal is met.

Every individual, whether under a ketogenic diet or not, must have answers to all the frequently asked questions. This will make it easy to avoid their associated side effects.

Finally, if you enjoyed this book, please take the time to share your thoughts and post a review on Amazon. It would be greatly appreciated! Thank you and good luck!

www.ingramcontent.com/pod-product-compliance
Lightning Source LLC
Chambersburg PA
CBHW060151290526
45789CB00003B/1002